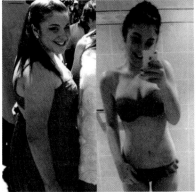
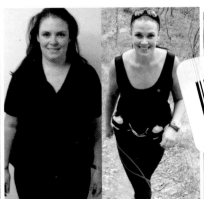

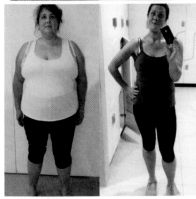

TOTAL
BODY
TRANSFORMATION

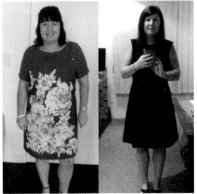

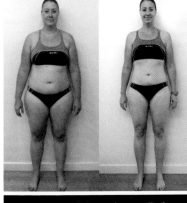

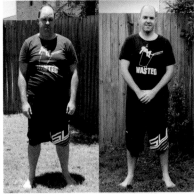

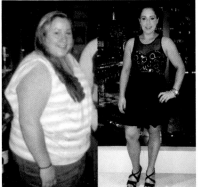

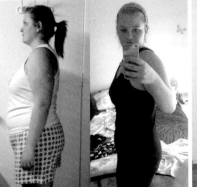

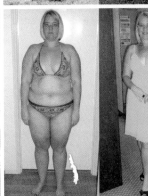

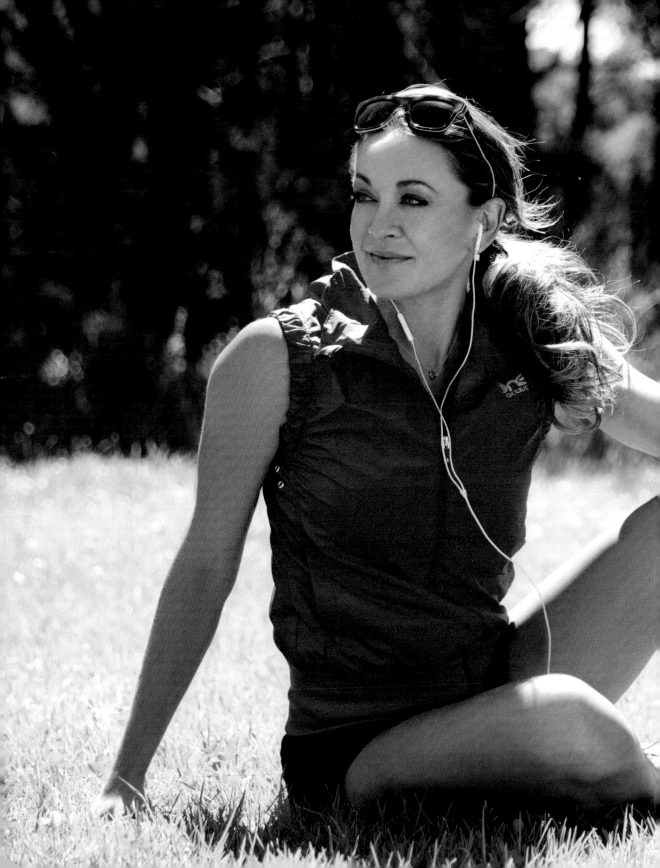

TOTAL BODY
TRANSFORMATION

Lose Weight Fast— and Keep It Off Forever!

michelle bridges

Ballantine Books

New York

This is a work of nonfiction. Some names have been changed.

A Zinc Ink Trade Paperback Original

Copyright © 2014 by Moore Bridges Nominees Pty Limited as trustee for the Moore Bridges Family Trust

Published in the United States by Zinc Ink, an imprint of Random House, a division of Random House LLC, a Penguin Random House Company, New York.

BALLANTINE and the HOUSE colophon are registered trademarks of Random House LLC.

ZINC INK is a trademark of David Zinczenko.

Exercise and lifestyle photography by Henryk Lobaczewski

Grateful acknowledgment is made to Penguin Group (Australia) for permission to reprint the following: from *Losing the Last 5 Kilos* by Michelle Bridges, photos on pages 4 and 45 by Robert Palmer, copyright © 2011 by Robert Palmer, and photos on pages 166 and 194 by Nick Wilson, copyright © 2011 by Nick Wilson; from *Crunch Time* by Michelle Bridges, food photography and recipes copyright © 2009 by Penguin Australia. All material reprinted by permission of Penguin Australia.

ISBN 978-0-553-39260-9
eBook ISBN 978-0-553-39261-6

Printed in the United States of America on acid-free paper

www.ballantinebooks.com

987654321

Book design by Mary A. Wirth
Spot illustrations: © istockphoto.com

To every one of the thousands of people

from all over the world who have trusted me

to help change their lives—

I have learnt so much from you!

You are my inspiration!

contents

introduction

I'm here for you

You are just a few small steps away from a new path to weight loss, better health, and overall improvement in the quality of your life—a path that you'll complete in just twelve weeks!

How can I make such a heady claim? Because I've already delivered on that very promise to tens of thousands of people just like you in my home country, Australia, and now I've updated and improved this time-tested, science-based plan just for you. Within just a few days of working together, through this program, you and I are going to become new best friends.

But who am I? Glad you asked!

For the better part of the past decade I've been the lead trainer on the Australian edition of *The Biggest Loser,* during which time I've been fortunate enough not just to impact the lives of my team members but to change the lives of the many thousands of Aussies who have read my seven books in print and followed my online 12 Week Body Transformation, or 12WBT. Through my incredible program, Australia has shed over 2 million pounds to date. I feel so proud and privileged to be able to play a part in helping people achieve their goals and live happier, healthier lives.

As I've published my books and connected with my online community, I have been so inspired by the stories of men and women turning their lives around, embracing the pleasures and joys (and challenges!) of a healthy diet and regular exercise. The more I've traveled, meeting people who have made positive changes in their lives, the more convinced I am that taking control of your body is the way not just to a healthier life, but to a happier life.

Over recent years, America, much like Australia, has grown, rather literally, to become one of the most overweight countries on earth. A combination of an overall lack of physical activity and an explosion in fast-food consumption has presented weighty challenges for all of us. The good news is that it's within our power to do something about it. There has never been a better time to get

real, get moving, and change our bodies—and in doing so, change our lives.

When it comes to weight loss and fitness, there are no must-follow rules. Nothing is set in stone. My goal is to plot a path forward for you, but one that easily adapts to the unique circumstances of your life. The most important thing you can do to improve your mind, body, and health is to believe—truly believe—that the power to make change happen is within you. From the very first moment you make a healthy choice over an unhealthy one, you are improving yourself. Making active decisions about the food you eat and the amount of exercise you do will transform your body, your energy levels, your outlook, and your future.

You've bought this book because you feel the need for change. I'm going to help you make it. Whether you want to lose 10 pounds or 100 pounds, this book will show you how. It's going to be hard work, but if you commit to the workouts and follow the nutrition plan you *will* see drastic changes in your body—dropping 10, 20, 25 pounds or more over the next few months, while improving your mood and dramatically slashing your risk from our biggest health threats. But only *you* can make the change—the book can't do it. I can't do it. No one can do it except you.

This kind of dramatic change will take you well out of your comfort zone, but let me ask you something: which discomfort would you prefer? The "I hate the way I look, I can't fit into anything, and I feel like crap" kind, or the "I'd better get my sneaks on and take the dog for a run and tonight I'll have grilled fish with no alcohol for dinner" kind? Which of these scenarios is *really* the most uncomfortable?

Once you have the nutrition and the exercise in place, weight loss is an exercise in mathematics; for most of us it's pretty much calories in versus calories out. But *The Biggest Loser* taught me that you *cannot* expect to lose weight and keep it off if you're still carrying emotional baggage. If you do not deal with the psychological aspect of weight loss, the physical just isn't going to happen.

In the first section, "Let's Begin!," I will help you get your head sorted out so you can address the emotional issues behind your struggle with health, fitness, and your weight. Let me tell you, most people don't struggle emotionally because they are overweight; they become overweight because they are busy fighting emotional battles. If you are going to find the solution to managing your weight permanently, then all the diet and exercise books in the world won't help unless you reprogram the way you think about food, exercise, and ultimately yourself.

In the second section, "Let's Train!," I will guide you through a series of killer workouts. I have worked in the fitness industry nearly all my life and I know the best exercises for rapid weight loss. But I'm not going to lie to you—in most cases it took *years* for you to put the weight on, so it's going to take real guts and determination to lose it. You absolutely must follow the exercise and nutrition plan for at least twelve weeks. Some of you will reach your goal weight before twelve weeks, others may need to continue for a few extra weeks, but whatever your individual needs, this program works!

In "Let's Get Cooking!," I show you how to minimize calories and maximize your eating. There is no way on this planet that you can accelerate yourself to lean and mean unless you put in some time in the kitchen, so I've included some of my favorite recipes.

I'm here to help you find the real you—the person who knows what you want and knows how to get it. You'll be your own personal trainer with this book, but you won't be alone. Let me lay it on the line for you: Your struggles are my struggles. Your demons are my demons. I have battled with my weight just as you have. But I will not tell you only what you want to hear. I will give it to you straight, because I am standing right there beside you in this. *I understand*. But what I want from you in exchange for this empathy is your trust and commitment.

No more excuses.

No more laying the blame at someone else's feet.

No more lying to yourself. It's time to be true to you. And I will be here, every step of the way, to guide you through it.

Let's rock!

"show me someone who put the weight back on because they lost it too quickly, and i'll show you five people who put the weight back on because they lost it too slowly!"

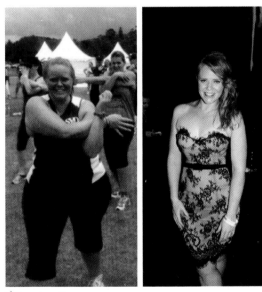

Elizabeth
You're 12 weeks away from a slimmer, sexier you.

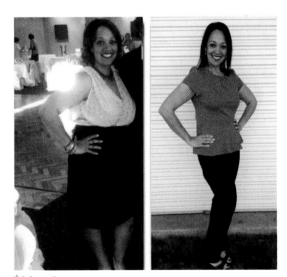

Wendy
Before: 213 pounds   After: 147 pounds

"Thank you for changing my life."

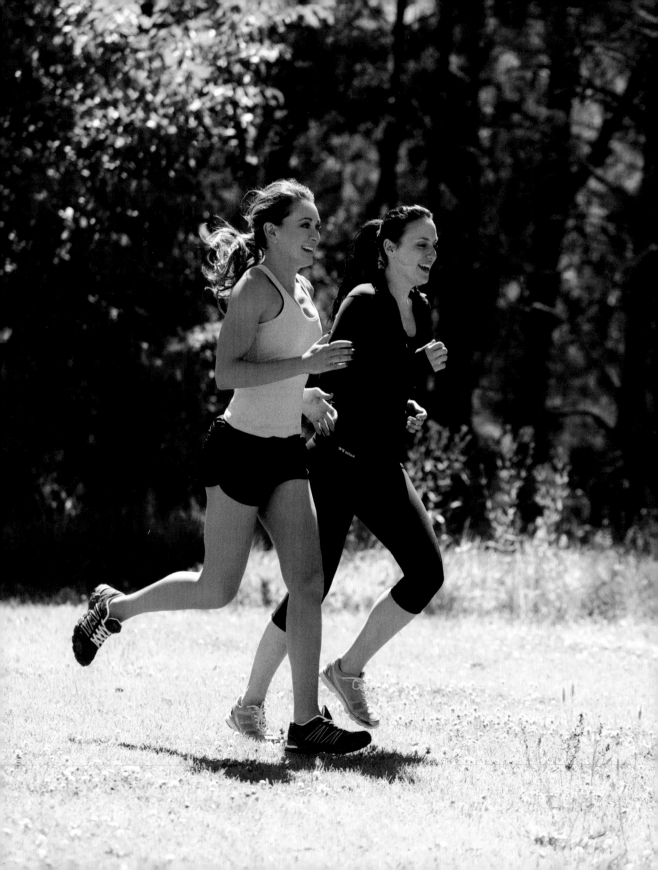

let's begin!

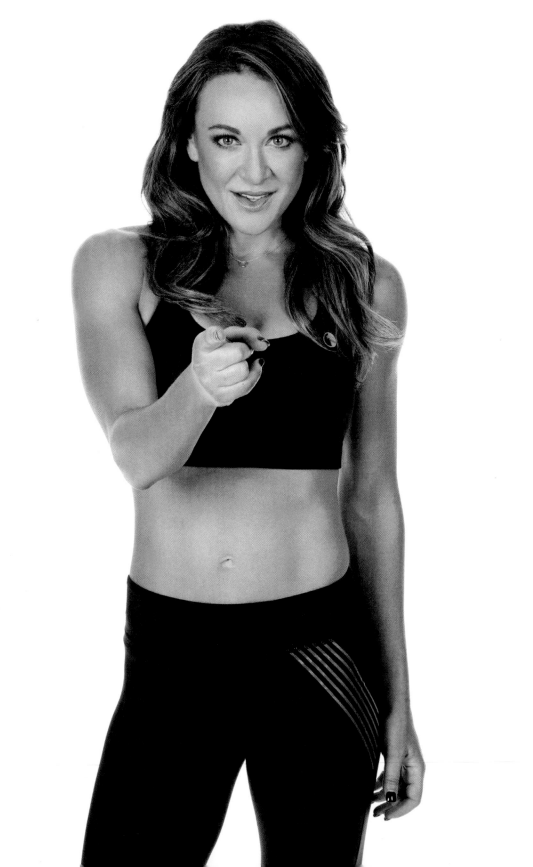

1

no more excuses!

"taking weight off is science, but keeping it off is psychology."

It's time to give up the excuses, people! You know—the ones you've been dragging out for so long that you actually believe them, and that you've managed to get everyone around you to believe, too!

If you hear your wife/husband/friends/kids saying, "She's always struggled with her weight, her parents were both big people," or "He'd love to exercise but he's got a bad back," then you can safely assume that you've done the perfect sell job. By enrolling others in your denial, you've avoided facing up to uncomfortable issues, or even quietly blamed these people as being part of the problem. You've built a world for yourself where no one is acknowledging what's real.

Here are some excuses I hear quite a bit—do any of them sound familiar?

- "I can't exercise because I have a sore knee."
- "I'm too busy to eat breakfast."
- "I can't cook healthy food because my husband/kids won't eat it."
- "Being big-boned runs in my family."
- "I'm too tired to go to the gym at night."

Maybe some of the excuses are based around finance: you know, "I can't afford a gym membership or a personal trainer," or "Healthy food is too expensive." Financial imperatives can be tricky because they can be hard to ignore. (When you're looking at financial excuses, make sure you compare the cost in real dollars. Prescription meds, lost days of work, health care costs . . . the price of being overweight is real!)

transformation story!

After my marriage I went from being fit and lean to fluctuating between 10 and 20 pounds over my ideal weight. I kept hoping that my one session a week with my personal trainer would magically get me back to my ideal weight. When I started to dislike looking in the mirror and refusing to have my photo taken, I realized it was time to take action.

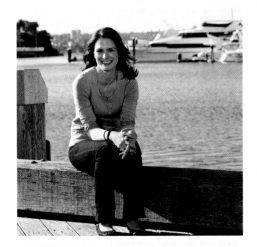

Sarah Visser

Thanks to Michelle's program, I finally found the focus and drive that had been missing over the past five years. I unlearned old habits, set firm goals to achieve, and stopped making excuses not to exercise. In twelve weeks I lost almost 20 pounds and am honestly the fittest, healthiest, and happiest I have ever been.

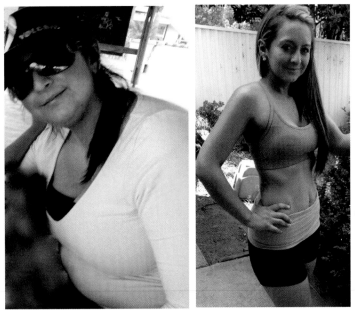

Jayne
Half her size!

However, the excuse that I hear the most is "I'm too busy." It gets dragged out by everyone, and therein lies a pertinent fact: *we are all busy*. People who are regular exercisers are busy. People who never exercise are busy. Very few of us would feel we have enough free time to stroll casually down to the gym for a workout or even to take a jog. But interestingly, often the busiest people in our society are the ones who exercise the most.

I work with many women who believe that making time for exercise amounts to putting themselves before their family, yet are resentful and angry that they are at "the bottom of the list." I ask them, "If your priority is your family, doesn't it make more sense to offer them a 'better' version of yourself? Wouldn't they prefer a mom who is happy, confident, and energized, rather than a tidy house?"

We're all busy. Your task is to make exercise part of your everyday life, just like brushing your teeth and making your bed. How badly do you want to do it? My grandpa used to say, "You can always find another hour in the day if you set the alarm clock an hour earlier!" It might mean you need to go to bed instead of sitting up and watching late-night TV—which, by the way, isn't going to get you *any* closer to your goal.

playing the victim

Cast your mind back to when you were a small child. Did you ever burst into tears to make people feel sorry for you so that you could get your own way? If it worked, and if you repeated it enough, it became a behavior pattern that you could potentially use for the rest of your life.

When you hear yourself coming out with comments like "It's okay for her, she's naturally slim" or "If only I didn't have the kids, I could exercise" then the "victim" alarm bells should be ringing, especially if you take your victimhood to the next level by seeming really upset. Your distress will ensure that others do not challenge your excuses, and you get to stay in your old patterns.

As a victim, you'll also have "villains"—the people or things you believe are "responsible" for your poor diet and exercise. It's only when you stop blaming people or circumstances for your unhappiness that you can empower

"talking is good, but it should set the stage for action, not become a replacement for it."

yourself to create the new you. There is no room for victims on my team.

you decide your future

Now I want you to think about a time in your past when you realized how unhappy you were with your weight, health, and fitness. It might be last week or it could go right back to your childhood. Take a moment to really reflect on this time in your life, and recall how you felt. Was it connected with a particular event or with disparaging remarks from others? Recall other, similar defining moments, even the ones you hoped to forget. Roll them around in your mind. How did you feel? What decision did you make about yourself? What self-limiting beliefs did you form? Stop, close your eyes, and take a few minutes with this.

Now, here's the clincher. The beliefs you formed about yourself in the past dictate your behavior today. And unless you're prepared to make a change in the present, your future can only reflect your past.

Your future needs to be decided *now,* and to do that you must ask yourself some questions about what you want. What kind of future would excite, move, and inspire you? If you wish to have that future, what are you prepared to change *right now*?

what is really holding you back?

If you've been to this place in the past but freeze up when you get to the part about making a change, you need to ask yourself, "What is holding me back?" Maybe you get "analysis paralysis" and overanalyze to the extent that it all becomes too complex and you become overwhelmed. Or maybe you simply don't know if you have the strength to do it. And before you know it, all the negative self-talk and the tired excuses flood back in and you shelve the whole idea: "I'll get to that next week/month/year." We all want it right now, but achieving it starts with action, not words.

Some people say they want to lose weight desperately, but they never convert their intentions into actions. Is this you? If it is, I want you to ask yourself what is it that you are afraid of. What is it about action that scares you?

"unless you're prepared to make a change in the present, your future can only reflect your past."

"most people don't struggle emotionally because they're overweight—they become overweight because they're struggling with emotions."

- Are you afraid of change? Of not being able to eat all the food you eat now? Well, my answer to that is simple: what the hell is so scary about that? You're clearly not starving! And I promise you, your new eating habits will help you lose weight *and* save you time and money.
- Does the thought of exercise send you into a blind panic? We're talking profound, life-extending change here, so it's definitely not time to be scared! *Please!* Exercise is nothing to be afraid of. Earthquakes, accidents, and war, yes; exercise, no.
- Or are you scared to fail? That's an easy one. The greatest opportunities for learning happen through screw-ups, especially if you are ready and willing to learn from them.

Sometimes when I'm talking to people who are struggling with their weight, it's as if they think that as long as they keep *talking* about weight loss, it will somehow magically happen. Talking is good, but it should set the stage for action, not become a replacement for it. It has to lead to something. Remember: thoughts, words, *action*!

If any of these fears ring true for you, then you need to face up squarely to them—bring them out into the open. Because when you acknowledge something, that's the first step to owning it and, in doing so, taking responsibility for it. You will no longer be able to put the blame on others or use all those well-honed excuses. *You* are in charge of the new you.

Why get up for that morning jog?

- Because your mind and your body will function better for it.
- Because you'll probably live quite a bit longer.
- Because you'll be less likely to live your later years with chronic disability, draining the emotions and finances of those around you.
- Because you won't be one of those resentful moms/dads/wives/husbands/partners who feel like they never get time for themselves (ouch!).
- But most important of all, you will be healthier *and* happier. (Many, *many* studies prove the effectiveness of exercise in managing depression.)

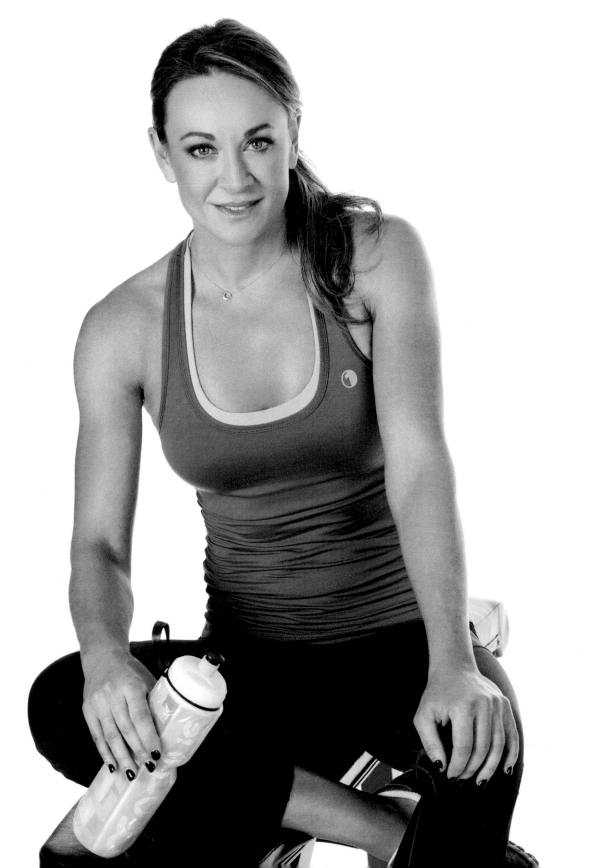

2

meet your metabolism

"the metabolism is the engine that drives the body."

"it must be my metabolism . . ."

I often hear people talking about fast and slow metabolisms. You know the kind of chat: "Oh, my husband can eat anything and he never puts on weight, he's got such a fast metabolism," or "I've got a really slow metabolism. I only have to look at a hamburger to put on two pounds." Now let's take this apart.

Put simply, our metabolic rate determines how quickly or slowly we convert the food we eat into the fuel that allows our bodies to perform actions: not just running, mowing the lawn, and playing with the kids, but basic bodily functions such as breathing, growing new cells, and perspiring. Even the action of digesting food requires energy.

So what determines our metabolic rate? There is a genetic component, of course, plus our age, and whether we live in a cold or warm climate. However, it's *the amount of lean muscle* we carry that will have the most profound effect on our metabolism—that, and the amount of fat we carry. Add some muscle, drop some fat, and our metabolic rate goes up. It isn't that complicated. In fact, it's pretty simple. *Our metabolic rates are largely determined by our lifestyles.*

Alarm bells start ringing whenever I hear that "groundbreaking scientific discoveries" are said to have unraveled the mystery of why we're all getting fat. These discoveries usually have three characteristics in common: first, you don't have to actually do any exercise to lose weight; second, they are complex and use a lot of big words; and third, (and here's the clincher) you usually have to buy something or you'll never learn the "secret" to avoiding a lifetime of self-loathing and fatness.

I reckon I'm a bit of a scientist. In fact, my time training people has been like one huge experiment. I've spent thousands of hours training hundreds and hundreds of people. All kinds of people: fat people, thin people, old people. And I'm here to tell you that *I* have discovered the secret! The secret that has eluded generations of scientists, intellectuals, and academics . . .

eat less.
move more.

Pretty complex, eh?

By eating less, I don't mean starving yourself. If you starve yourself, you *will* lose weight, but your body is biologically geared to switch to survival mode when there is less food around, and that lowers your metabolism by eating away at your precious muscle mass as well as your fat stores.

my top four metabolism boosters

Now that you understand how a sluggish metabolism is a key reason why it's so hard to lose the last 10 pounds, I want to take you through my top four diet and exercise tips for *boosting* your metabolism.

1. eat regularly

This is important. Your metabolism slows down when you sleep because you are *not eating* and cranks up again when you eat a good breakfast. Since your metabolism slows down without food, it makes sense to eat regularly during the day, but *what* you eat is critical. If your three meals a day are interspersed with crappy, high-calorie snacks, you will be defeating the purpose.

Starting the day with a good breakfast also stops you from playing games with yourself: "If I skip breakfast and have an apple for lunch, I'm allowed to gorge myself when I get home." My mantra is: "Eat like a king for breakfast, a prince for lunch, and a pauper for dinner." Take in calories when you need them.

2. drink water

Apart from being an appetite suppressant, water is also essential for efficient kidney and liver function. These guys are responsible for breaking down and disposing of the waste products that you generate as you lose weight, and if there isn't enough water in your system, your liver and kidneys will try to source water from elsewhere in your body, drying out your skin, muscles, connective tissue, and other organs in the process—a recipe for disaster.

Water actually boosts your metabolism, as your body has to expend energy warming it in your stomach so that it can be absorbed. But don't get too excited and start carrying around a thermos of iced spring water. Drinking a bottle of water only expends 25 calories, about the equivalent of either a carrot or a walnut.

3. eat metabolism-boosting foods

Your body actually expends energy digesting, absorbing, and storing food. This is referred to as the "thermal effect" of food. Now before you get too carried away with the notion of gorging yourself and shrinking away in the process, you need to be aware that the thermal effect of food accounts for only 5–10 percent of your total daily calorie expenditure. By far the biggest calorie-burning factor is your basal metabolic rate (the energy required to keep your body functioning), which accounts for 65–75 percent of your daily calorie expenditure. The remaining 15–30 percent is accounted for by physical activity. Now, that's not just going to the gym or going for a run. It's *all* of your physical activity—folding the laundry, brushing your teeth, even scratching your bum.

how much water?

We're constantly told that we should drink eight glasses of water per day, but this is misleading. Does a 300-pound man need the same amount of water as a 120-pound woman? No. And besides, what's a glass? The truth is we need less than a half ounce of water per pound of body weight per day. An average teacup holds 8 oz and a water bottle 20 oz. I weigh 130 pounds, so I'm going to need three bottles of water, or a couple of bottles of water and a couple of cups of tea, to be roughly where I need to be.

Your body digests different foods at different rates, with simple carbohydrates (including sugar and refined grains) being the quickest. Protein is digested the slowest, thereby expending the most energy. Fats are digested after carbs and before protein, and are converted directly to—you guessed it—fat.

Grains, vegetables, fruits, and other fibrous foods are unrefined carbohydrates and are digested slowly, keeping your insulin levels steady and avoiding an insulin spike. This is important, because insulin is a hormone that tells your body to *store* fat.

Fish and shellfish are great choices, along with sea vegetables (kelp, seaweed). These foods are rich in iodine, which helps to keep your thyroid gland healthy. An underactive thyroid can lead to weight gain, depression, and general misery so make sure there's iodine in your diet. If you're not keen on seafood, it's also present in iodized salt (no surprise there), eggs, and dairy products.

Fish has the added advantage of being a rich source of omega-3 fats, essential fatty acids (these are "essential" because our bodies can't manufacture them and we have to get them from our food). One of the groovy things that omega-3 fats do is to regulate a hormone called *leptin,* which plays a major role in deciding how hungry you get and whether your body will burn fat or store it. Now *that's* a protein I want to take to lunch!

Low-fat yogurt, milk, and cheese are definitely on the menu because they're packed full of calcium, which some studies have found can crank up your metabolism.

4. focus on strength-training exercises

I love aerobic exercise. I can safely report that if you're looking for a great workout, a killer calorie burn, and more feel-good happiness than a dance party, then you can't beat a solid 40-minute aerobic exercise session to get your heart rate up and your waist mea-

surement down. All that puffing and panting somehow seems actually enjoyable when you're staring down the finish line of a good cardio workout.

But does it increase your metabolism? The short answer is yes, but *you will need to go hard.* Ramp up the intensity and you will see an improvement, but it will only last as long as the workout. Aerobic exercise does not build lean muscle mass, which is the principal determining factor of your basal metabolic rate.

After exercise, our bodies need to get back to their normal resting state—a bit like cleaning up after a party. This includes building molecules and repairing cells, returning hormone levels to normal, developing our nervous system to accommodate any changes that have taken place, and relocating the free fatty acids in our bloodstream, to name a few. All this takes energy, and that energy is sourced from increased oxygen intake *after* you've finished training. This "afterburn" is known as excess post-exercise oxygen consumption (EPOC) and can last anywhere from three to sixteen hours after your workout, depending on what kind of exercise you were doing, how hard you were doing it, and how long you were doing it for.

Now, before you start bombarding me with emails wanting to know which exercises maximize afterburn, I have to tell you that it's not 100 percent clear. This is because it's difficult to compare the different types of exertion. However, I do know that although the EPOC effect is greater with weight training (anaerobic exercise) than aerobic exercise, aerobic exercise does use more calories *during* the session.

You could argue that weight training has the added benefit of increasing your muscle mass, thereby increasing your metabolic rate, which would be true. But keep it real: 2 pounds of muscle will add 10–20 calories to your basal metabolic rate, and as any weight trainer will tell you, it takes a *lot* of work to put on 2 pounds of muscle.

There is another excellent side effect of exercise: our skeletal muscles become more sensitive to insulin, the hormone that shuttles sugar out of the bloodstream and into the muscles for energy (good) or into the fat cells (bad). This means that our body doesn't have to produce as much, and so there's less of it floating around in our bloodstream. Too much insulin in our bloodstream means there is more of it to act on our fat cells to take up glucose and make even *more* fat. So exercise not only burns fat but also helps to stop our bodies from making more. Exercise rocks for *so* many reasons.

The other thing that exercise does is to help lower our stress levels. It does that by reducing our levels of *cortisol*. This hormone is actually quite important to our everyday functioning, and isn't only secreted in stressful situations. It's involved in glucose metabolism and blood sugar maintenance, our inflammatory response, regulation of our blood pressure, and maintenance of our immune function.

It's during times of stress, however, that our adrenal glands are pumping this stuff out by the bucketload. It's this "fight-or-flight" hormone that gives us a burst of energy, heightens memory functions, and several other stress-related changes. The problem is, our modern way of life means that our cortisol levels get pumped up so many times during our busy days that they don't get much of a chance to return to normal. And one of the things an elevated cortisol level does is to increase our level of abdominal fat, the most dangerous fat repository of all, because of the increased risk for diabetes, cardiovascular disease, hypertension, and certain cancers associated with visceral fat.

Exercise, however, *reduces* our cortisol levels, which is one of the reasons we feel de-stressed after a good workout, which in turn reduces fat deposits. Good, eh?

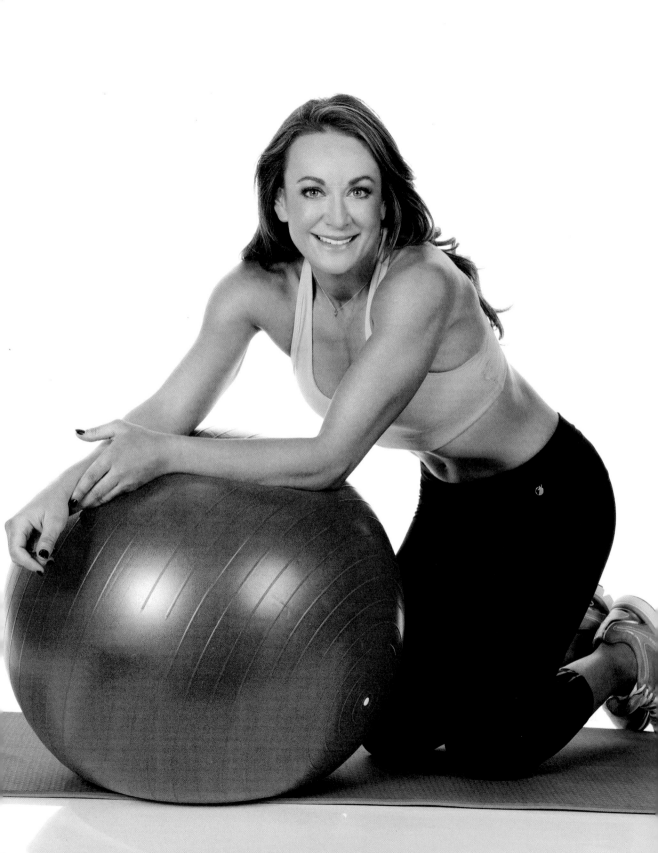

3

mind...set!

"you've gotta believe to achieve."

how our minds work against us (and how to change that)

You'll hear many elite athletes attest that while their training is no walk in the park, the biggest factor in determining their success had to do with their way of thinking. The right mind-set is absolutely critical for success in any physical endeavor, whether it's hitting a home run, winning a footrace, or dropping 20 pounds.

When I first begin working with my weight loss clients, the great majority tell me that they feel they have "lost control"—and not just of their eating habits. They say they have lost control of their weight, their exercise patterns, and their lives in general. Later, when they've lost weight and regained their health

and fitness, they say the *exact opposite*: "I feel so much better in myself, so much more in control." They are firmly planted in the driver's seat. These people haven't just exercised their bodies, they've also exercised their minds.

Remember—get your head right, and your body will follow.

the excuses

Our bad habits (poor food choices, little exercise, emotional eating) thrive on a huge array of colorful excuses. Do you:

- Tell yourself you'll feel better if you eat something when you feel emotional, whether you are hungry or not?
- Find excuses for not exercising ("It's too cold" or "My ankle is sore")?

- Find excuses for making poor food choices ("My children hate vegetables" or "I don't have anything in the fridge")?

types of excuses

There are three basic types of excuses, and identifying which types you're making is the first step to challenging them and coming up with new habits and behaviors.

1. internal excuses

These are based around the old internal negotiation:

"I'm a bit tired tonight, so I won't train in case I hurt myself."

"I've fallen off the wagon, so what's the point?"

"I'm not motivated. I'll wait and get a training partner to fire me up."

"I am too unfit at the moment. I'll get myself back in shape, then I'll go back to the gym." (I love that one!)

2. external excuses within your control

These are based around external factors over which you do have some control but which you choose to allow to control you. For example:

"I'm really busy at work at the moment."

"It's cold/wet outside and I might catch a cold."

"It's too expensive at my local gym."

"My training buddy can't make it tonight."

3. external excuses out of your control

These are out-of-the-blue events that affect your training or nutrition, such as a car accident, a sick child, or a family crisis. Clearly you have no control over these situations, but once they have been resolved, make sure you get straight back into your training and healthy eating. When it comes to rocky times, I've found my training to be my savior.

Once you work out the kind of excuses you're using to prevent yourself from eating right and training well, you can organize the mental ammo you will need to challenge them. Look at the example on the next page and then draw up a list of your ten favorite excuses and your solutions.

Challenging your excuses takes willpower, and each time you exercise that willpower, the stronger it becomes. All you're doing is replacing old habits with new ones. And don't give me any rubbish about how hard it

excuse	type	solution
"I'm really busy at work at the moment, so I can't go to the gym."	External	Organize your days so you *can* fit in your training. Tell yourself you deserve the break and that you will be more efficient and focused at work if you exercise.
"I'm a bit tired tonight, so I won't train in case I hurt myself."	Internal	Do it anyway. If you train, you'll get stronger with less chance of injury, plus you'll sleep better.
"It's too cold/wet outside for training and I might catch a cold."	External	Wear a hoodie, plus you'll soon warm up with exercise.
"I'm not motivated. I'll wait until I get a training partner to fire me up."	Internal	You have to learn to fly solo. The only way to do it is to do it. The key is consistency, not motivation.
"It's too expensive at my local gym."	External	Find another one near work, or start with running, cycling, or some other training that doesn't cost money.

is to learn new habits when you are older, either. That's just another excuse. Our brains are *wired* for challenges—they thrive on learning new stuff, and there's more and more research around to show that as we get older, we gotta use it or lose it. So keep coming up with alternatives. For example:

- When you feel emotional, instead of opening the fridge, do something else (go for a walk, call a friend).

- When you hear yourself looking for excuses not to exercise, put on your trainers and just do it.

- Outmaneuver your weaknesses (put fresh veggies in your fridge, don't have chocolate in the house).

the denial

Remember the old saying: what we resist persists. The more we try to ignore or deny something, the bigger it becomes. You *know* you should be cooking instead of getting takeout, or doing your training instead of crashing in front of the television. The longer you put it off, the harder it seems.

By *choosing* the harder option you strengthen your resolve, your inner confidence, and your self-belief.

One of my contestants told me about a brilliant method she used that she called the layaway system or the "cooling-off" period. If she saw some chocolate she wanted to eat, she would "put it on layaway" for twenty-four hours. If after twenty-four hours she still wanted it, she would eat it and then work it into her calorie count for the day. If she didn't want it, she'd just let it go.

By saying no the first time and walking away, she was taking responsibility for her choice, and that was empowering. She wasn't telling herself that she *couldn't* have the chocolate, just that she would control *when* she could have it. But get this—saying no the first time made her resolve even stronger, so the next day she usually found herself saying no again. Cool, huh?

When you boil it all down, she had simply learned a new behavior. How? She first changed the *story* she told herself. Instead of saying, "I can't control myself—I just have to eat this now," she said, "I can choose when I eat this. I'm going to put this on layaway."

the negative self-talk

To help you ditch your unhealthy habits around food and exercise, you'll also need to bust a few myths about yourself that you've been dragging around for years. Stories like "I have the willpower of a Labrador retriever" or "I always end up chucking it in because I don't have any self-control."

I believe in the power of language, so if you are saying these things out loud and in your head day in and day out, guess what? That's right—you are putting these negative messages out there to the universe big-time. If you say them, you believe them and you are *making them happen.*

The truth is that *none* of these negative opinions is true. Why? Because, you've almost always constructed these self-limiting thoughts in moments when emotion was running high and you weren't thinking clearly.

More than likely, you made a decision to go on a diet or health kick on a whim, in the heat of the moment: after a fight, after a binge, or after you spent three hours getting ready for an event you didn't end up going to because you felt like a fat cow and so you burst into tears and consoled yourself with a family-size block of chocolate. Then, with the decision made to get stuck into a diet and exercise regimen, you proceeded to go about it for approximately three or four days, after which time you kinda ran out of emotional steam, and hey, it was your dad's birthday and you just felt too rude to say no to a piece of Black Forest cake.

Then, bang, you've proved to yourself once again that you have the willpower of iceberg lettuce and you tell yourself that losing weight is forever out of your reach.

Right?

Wrong!

The problem is that you set your goal when you were feeling vulnerable and emotional. Your decision to lose weight must be genuine and unemotional.

mind training

In the same way that our muscles become stronger and more efficient when we train them, our minds do, too. I've given you some ways to challenge your excuses, denial, and negative self-talk, but there are two other powerful tools that I use all the time, both for myself and for my clients: goal setting and consistency.

1. set your goals

Goals give you focus, but you must work out *how* you will get there. Your goals need to be SMART.

S Specific. No fluffy stuff—be crystal clear about where you're going. For example, "I'm joining a gym today."

M Measurable. Get all the cold, hard numbers so you can monitor your progress: get on the scale, take your measurements, try on your skinny clothes, calculate your BMI (see page 35), see your doctor and get your blood pressure and cholesterol readings.

A Achievable. Your goal needs to be one that you are capable of reaching given your available time, job and family commitments, and so on.

R Realistic. Similar to achievable, but a notch higher. For example, "I'm going to lose 40 pounds in the next twelve weeks" is realistic (especially if you are morbidly obese), but "I'm going to lose 40 pounds in the next three weeks" is not, unless you plan to lose a leg in an unfortunate shark attack.

T Time-based. Once you've set your goal weight, then you need to draw up a day-by-day, week-by-week plan and execute it with precision. For example, "I will lose 40 pounds in twelve weeks, which is about 3.3 pounds per week."

2. be consistent

Of all the questions that I am asked about exercise and healthy living (and God knows there are plenty to choose from: what to eat, when to train, whether to stretch, whether to do weights or cardio), there is one that endlessly haunts me: "So tell me, Michelle, how do you stay motivated?" When I hear it, I want to tear my hair out, because what I do is not about motivation, it's about consistency. Motivation is about *feeling*—determined, enthusiastic, frenzied, even angry—and is therefore fickle and unreliable. You can't count on it being there. Consistency, however, is about *doing*. Consistency isn't something that you need to wind up like a coiled spring every morning. You don't need to plug it in and recharge it every few hours. It is that steady yet relentless journey to an end. It doesn't require profound thought. You quite literally *just effing do it*. In fact, I have a T-shirt that makes the point a little more emphatically by boasting my favorite acronym on the front in bold letters: "J F D I."

When I've racked up a fifteen-hour day and I'm driving past the gym on the way home, do I feel *motivated*? When it's 40 degrees and raining outside and my alarm goes off at 5:00 a.m., do I feel *motivated*? Are you nuts? Sure—motivated to *stay in bed*!

So here are my tips for consistency:

1. Don't think, just *do*. Just put on your gym gear, head out the door, and get over it.

2. Don't start bargaining with yourself. No trade-offs—none of that "Maybe I could skip this morning and go for a run at lunchtime" bullshit. *Just get on with it.*

3. If you feel yourself wavering, apply the 10-minute rule. Do what you need to do—exercise, study, rehearse—for just 10 minutes. If you still don't feel like it after 10 minutes, then treat yourself by going back to bed. Trust me—it doesn't happen. In fact, some of my best workouts have come after I've applied the 10-minute rule for myself.

If you want to know my recipe for success, just read the T-shirt!

the power of language

Your choice of words has a lot more clout than you may think, and this applies as much to your self-talk as it does to your dialogue with others.

Have you ever heard an Olympian speak about her goals or a mountaineer interviewed before a major climb? Their language reflects their belief in themselves. It's positive and productive, and it's a skill that has taken them time to learn.

transformation story!
Go, Greg!

Greg, one of the contestants on Australia's *The Biggest Loser*, was constantly beating himself up about how he had let himself go and worrying that his wife would leave him if he didn't clean up his act—unless he died from obesity-related health issues first. Greg had also been an athlete in his youth, and it killed him that he had let himself slip so far from the healthy young man he used to be.

But he took back control and began an aggressive weight loss journey that saw him revert to his old athletic self, and with that came more positive language. Soon "I can't" and "I'm too tired" were replaced by "I can" and even "Get the hell out of my way because I'm coming through!"

He fired up not only himself but also the rest of the team. Interestingly, as his self-confidence returned, people really loved to be around him, including me. His positive outlook was infectious, and soon he had the crew; my co-star, Shannan Ponton; and the other team members hanging out with him. Everyone loves being around positive, uplifting people!

Negative self-talk is a habit that forms like any other unproductive habit. When did it start? Who knows! But I bet you didn't tell yourself you were a stupid, fat cow when you were a five-year-old. Back then I bet you thought you were invincible and ready to tackle the world! Granted, the world back then was kindergarten, but it doesn't matter, because it was *your* world.

Take the time to stop and listen to what you are saying, even when you think it's an off-the-cuff comment. We are so used to putting ourselves down that we don't even notice a put-down anymore. Particularly watch out for humor that disguises self-loathing, in comments such as "I might be a big guy, but there's a whole lot more of me to love" or "Look out! Big sista comin' through!"

I had a client whose email address was bigfatgirl@whatever.com—I'm not kidding. I had her change it immediately. She wasn't going to continually put it out to the universe that she was a big fat girl anymore.

How often do you hear "Oh, once I start eating I just can't stop. That's just the way I am"? That's crap, and you know it! That's you giving yourself permission to avoid taking responsibility for yourself, and you've said it so many times you think it's true. Grow up! That sentence and any others like it are now *gone*.

My friend Craig was constantly getting on

my case when I used the word *hopefully*, and not because he's a pessimist. In fact, he's the most amazingly positive person I know. Craig explained his thoughts to me about hope: "How is what you're saying you *want* to happen *going* to happen if you are only *hoping* it will happen? What has hoping got to do with anything? Okay, I am really, really, *really* hoping now, Mishy," and he would screw up his brow and try to stop giggling at the same time. Naturally I would slap him and tell him to shut up and stop being so right all the time.

How true is that, though? How many times do you hear yourself or others say, "Hopefully I'll be able to fit into those jeans by Christmas" or "Hopefully I will be able to get fit and lose weight by summer"?

Yeah, and I'm hoping for world peace! Take *hope* out of your vocabulary and replace it with words denoting action, not aspiration. Say "I will be two pounds lighter by the end of this week" instead of "I hope I lose two pounds this week."

I reckon we do it as a backstop. "I'll use the word *hope,* just in case I fail, and then I can say that I didn't really mind either way."

And while we're here, why are we so hung up on failure? I hate failing. It totally sucks. But I have learned some major lessons through my failures, lessons that have made me more determined. Lessons I wouldn't have learned if I had succeeded. Not achieving what I set out to do certainly didn't kill me, and it made me appreciate achievement so much more.

At some point you've just got to go for it and say, "I am going to do this! And no minor setback is going to stop me." You must absolutely stand up and shout it to the world that you're a heat-seeking missile homing in on your destination. This is the attitude of people who achieve their goals. This is truly the path to success.

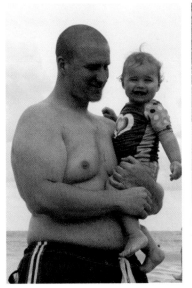 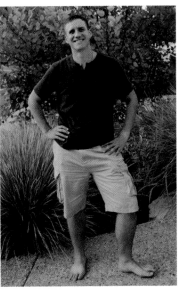

Dave
Finally the fit dad
his kids deserve.

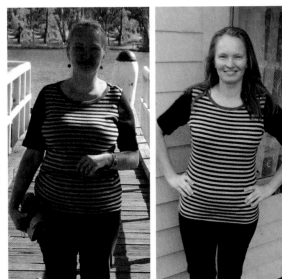

Urzula
"I hope my journey
can inspire others."

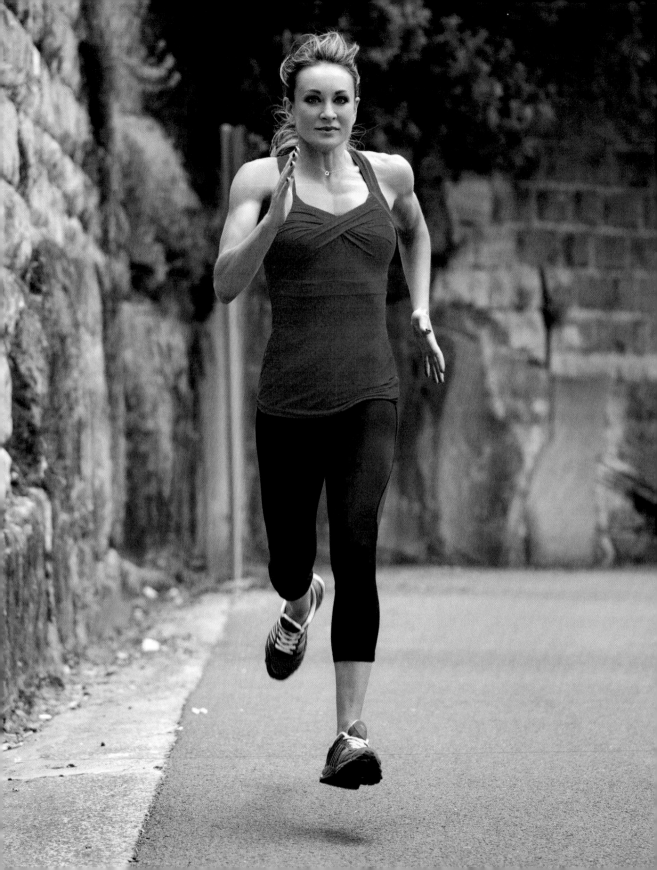

4

you gotta have a plan!

"it's knowing how you're going to get there that makes it happen."

Every great journey needs a map, and the best navigators are the ones who have considered all the parts of the journey. They take into account fuel, terrain, weather, equipment, and other factors such as communication in emergencies.

It's the same for you on your weight loss journey. If you are serious about making this happen, you need a game plan. And it's got to be realistic—by this I mean that you must acknowledge what you've got and how you can make the best of it. In other words, if you are small and heavy, you will not be able to get your body to look like something off the catwalk.

It's a tough call, particularly when we are bombarded with images of what "perfect" women and men are supposed to look like.

To some degree we are seeing a move away from this thinking, with role models who refuse to fall into line, who are happy with their bodies the way they are. But it's hard not to be weight-obsessed with media headlines like "Celebs' Fat Days," "Celebrity Beach Bodies," "Detox in Three Days," and "Seven Days to Washboard Abs." It's endless, and we *all* know it's bullshit, but we still let ourselves get sucked in. So get past aiming for the unachievable and just take these images for what they are—digitally altered pictures of pretty boys and girls who have just as many bad hair days as we do.

We tend to hate our body when we are struggling with our weight, and we must accept, embrace, and love our body because it's perfect as it is. You won't be able to move forward on your journey until you take this important step, so if you've been hating yourself, picking at your imperfections, beating yourself up about how you look, it's time to do the opposite and start loving your body because it's your body, and it's the only one you've got.

Think of it like this: you've hated your body for a while now, but has it helped? What if you did the opposite and started giving it a little love? I have all my clients say out loud, "I love myself and I love my body." I get them to say it to me until they *believe* it.

set your goal

The next step is to ask yourself what you really want. What is it that you are looking for? What is the life-changing result that you want to achieve? Is it only about weight loss? Or is it about fitness, too? Do you have some health issue that must be addressed, such as high cholesterol or high blood sugar levels? You need to be absolutely clear about your plan. And remember, it needs to be SMART. Remember: specific, measurable, achievable, realistic, and time-based.

The words *want* and *try* don't get used in SMART terminology. "I want to lose 40 pounds" means just that—you want to lose 40 pounds. "I'm going to lose 40 pounds" means just that—you *will* lose 40 pounds.

Now that you have a clear understanding of what you are aiming for, it's time to go get it!

1. get on the scale

Yep. That's right, you heard me. And if you don't have one, go and buy a good one and then come back to this spot. Your scale and tape measure are the tools of your trade because they're how you'll measure your success.

Take out a notebook and write down your weight, the day, and the time. You will weigh yourself at the end of each week at the same time.

2. get out the tape measure

Measure your chest, waist, hips, thighs, and arms. Try to be accurate, and also record *how* you made those measurements. It's *really* important to do it the same way each time, so if you have your partner or a friend helping you, try to use that same person again.

- **Chest.** Girls, run the tape measure right across your nipples with your bra on. (Guys, you can take your bra off!)
- **Waist.** Use your belly button as a guide.
- **Hips.** Measure your hips at the widest point.
- **Thighs.** Measure the distance from the

tip of your pelvic bone (iliac crest) down to the side of the knee joint. Halve the distance and mark that point on your leg with a pen. Now, wrap the tape around the mark. Do the same on the other leg.

- Arms. Measure from the tip of the shoulder joint down to the elbow. Halve the distance and draw a mark. Now wrap the tape around the mark to measure. Do the same on the other arm.

Next, measure your height, and along with your weight calculate your body mass index (BMI)—see page 35. This will give you a handle on where your weight *should* be.

3. take a photo of yourself

Now get a pair of jeans, preferably ones that are hard to zip up. Then choose a non-stretchy shirt or top that you're struggling to get into. These are your "benchmark clothes" and often work better as motivators than measurements do. Take a photo of yourself in them, and then take a photo of yourself in your underwear or bathing suit. (If you're sweating this, just remember *The Biggest Loser* contestants, who do it on national TV!)

4. get a calorie counter

You'll need it when you get to the end of this chapter. Don't bother complaining to me that calorie counting is no good—you absolutely have to know how much fuel you're taking on board, just as much as you need to know how much fuel you're burning. I mean, if you were going to drive on the interstate, would you really do it without knowing how much gas you have in the tank? Of course not! This journey is no different.

"But you can't expect me to remember all those numbers," I hear you say. Just check in on what you usually eat—we're creatures of habit, so there's usually only a dozen or so foods that we habitually buy. It's really not that complicated. And besides, weren't you the one saying, "I really want this! I really want to lose weight! And I'll do whatever it takes"?

5. make a calendar

Put together a large calendar and stick it up where you see it every day. Mark on it your target weight week by week, month by month, until you reach your goal weight. (See Chapter 5 for how to calculate your healthy body weight.) So if you're going to lose 50 pounds in twelve weeks, then your weight needs to be coming down by a bit more than 4 pounds per week.

But is this realistic? In my experience, if you weigh 285 pounds or more, you can expect to lose between 3 and 11 pounds per week, with the first few weeks showing the greatest losses. (One of my clients who weighed 360 pounds lost over 14 pounds in the first week!)

If your weight ranges from 220 to 285 pounds, you can lose around 3–7 pounds per week. If you are under 220 pounds, you'll usually drop between 1 and 3 pounds per week. Of course, much of this will depend on your commitment and determination, which will be tested when you have a week where you did not lose as much as you planned. Just *keep going* and reread "Be Consistent" on page 20.

your weight	expected weight loss per week
less than 220 lbs	1–3 lbs
220–285 lbs	3–7 lbs
more than 285 lbs	7–11 lbs

6. plan your daily workout time

Okay, this is the *big* one! This is the key to reaching the target weights you've marked on your calendar. It's time to go through your daily planner, because it's critical that you find the time to exercise. (See "Let's Train!" for all you need to know about your workouts.) Before you open your mouth, don't give me the old "I don't have enough time" excuse. That's crap and you know it. If you've

chosen to do this, this is the work you *must* do to make that change a reality. Maybe you need to be setting the alarm earlier. Morning training is not only great for being uninterrupted but also biochemically better for weight loss because your glycogen stores are depleted and your body *has* to source other energy stores (fat).

Once you've assigned your training time, book it in as an "appointment." That way when someone is trying to pull you out of it you can say, "Sorry, I have an appointment between 1:00 and 2:00 p.m., but I can see you after that." People aren't likely to ask you what kind of appointment you have, and if you tell them it's a workout, they will usually try to tell you that it's not that important, that you can just skip one, that you don't need to train, blah, blah, blah. They will project their own guilt about not exercising onto you, and we're not going to have negative people around us. So simply tell them that you have an appointment—it'll save a lot of time *and* will guarantee you get to your workout.

Be realistic about your time. If your job has got you behind your desk until 7:00 p.m. every day, then you may have to restructure your day so you can exercise either early in the morning or at lunchtime. Or put it to your boss that you will start earlier on the

> *"morning training is not only great for being uninterrupted but also biochemically better for weight loss."*

days that you want to leave earlier. If you have children, organize child care with the school, your partner, or family/friends. Or find a gym with a child care center if you have a preschooler.

7. get support

It's vital to have a network of close family and friends who are fully aware how important this is to you and who will support you. Don't skip this step. You absolutely must have an "enrollment conversation" with them. Make a time to get together with your closest family members where there will be no distractions. Call it a "family meeting," and make sure you have their full attention (no TV on in the background, and so on.).

This is where you are going to inspire them with your passion so that they can help you make positive and fulfilling changes to your health, your body, your fitness, your outlook, and ultimately your relationship with them. You need to blow them away with your honesty, courage, determination, and spirit, which will happen naturally if you speak from the heart. This conversation has two critical elements.

- You will be declaring to the people who are important to you that you are tidying up your physical and emotional well-being.
- You are enrolling those around you in your plans, helping to ensure your success.

Be brave! Go over the changes that you need to make with them—exercising, going to bed earlier so you can train in the mornings, and making changes in the food you'll be eating. Your passion will be infectious, and you may find others around you will want to join you in your goals. But whether they accept or reject your plan, welcome or disapprove of it, ultimately doesn't matter. This is about *you*.

My guess is that you'll probably be greeted with *shock* (especially if you are someone who never speaks about your weight), *tears* (it might be the first time you've gotten real with your family in a long time), and *respect* (because ultimately they love you). The bigger the emotions, the better!

Make an appointment to see your doctor for a full checkup—you'll need to record your vital stats (blood pressure, cholesterol level). I talk more about this on page 230.

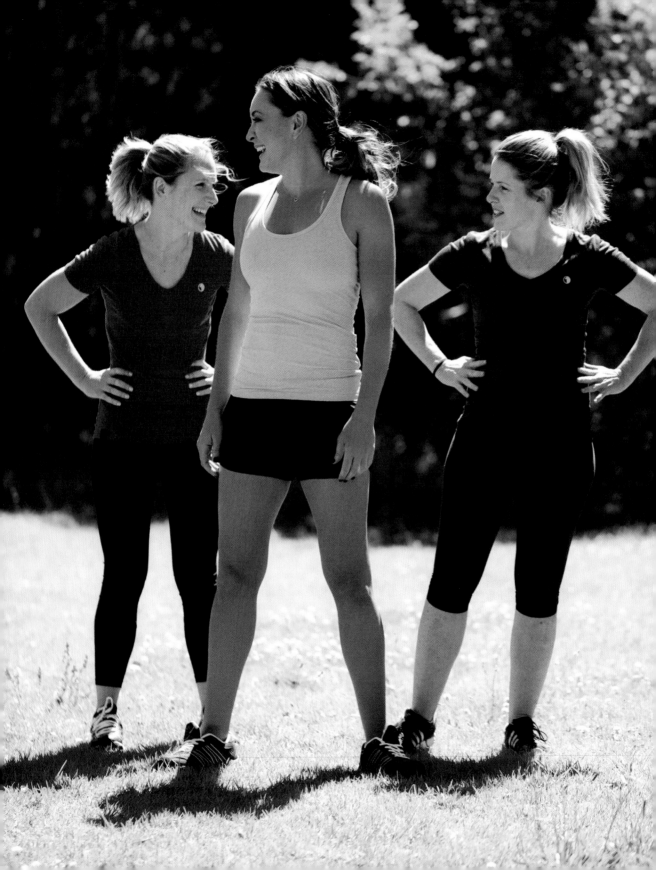

8. throw out all the crap food in your house

Get rid of all the sugary, processed foods in your pantry, fridge, and freezer. If you're not sure what has to go, have a look at Chapter 11. Then copy down my fridge, freezer, and pantry shopping lists from that chapter and go shopping. (Make sure you have had a healthy meal before you hit the supermarket!) This is another reason you need to have the enrollment conversation with the rest of your family, as it means you're less likely to get any bitching about what will no longer be found in the pantry. If the kids complain, remember that *you* are the adult. They can have what they want when they move out of your home, get a job, and pay their own way. Besides, as a parent, you have a responsibility to give your children the best possible start in the world, with healthy bodies, well-functioning brains, and a strong sense of self—not overweight, self-conscious, embarrassed, and facing a future with poor health and all the unhappiness and heartache that come with it. Setting up good nutritional habits is one of the best gifts you can give your children. This is the *new* you—now you're in control, you're in charge.

9. get a "new you" journal

This is a journal I use with my clients to keep the plan going and keep them on track. What does NEW stand for?

N   Nutrition. You'll write down everything you eat and drink. Be descriptive: white bread, whole-wheat bread, half-and-half, skim milk, and so on. Write down the calories and add them up at the end of each day and each week.

E   Emotion. You'll record how you are feeling emotionally each day. How did you feel when you woke up? Were you lethargic all day? Were you on fire all day? What was your "self-talk"?

W   Workout. You will fill in the details around not only your formal training session and how you felt during it but any incidental exercise you did as well. This is where you will log how many calories you burned off in your training sessions (see page 232).

This journal is your bible. It is the tangible reference to each step you take toward your goal. It is where you learn about your exercise: what's working, what isn't, where you train better (inside or outside, morning or evening), and how many calories you can burn in one session. It's where you learn about your calorie intake: are you eating too little during the day and too much at night? It's also where you learn about yourself and how these changes are affecting you mentally and emotionally. Download a template from my website (www.michellebridges.com) or use the version on page 232.

10. start a 7-day food diary

The first entry in your journal will be your measurements, followed by your 7-Day Food Diary. You must write down *everything* you eat and drink for one week. The descriptions of the food and the quantities need to be very detailed. For example: white bread, whole-wheat bread, or multigrain bread; heavy cream or soy milk; 1 cup of cooked brown rice; 16 oz skim latte, and so on. (See Richard's story on page 66 for a sample page in an *honest* 7-Day Food Diary.) The time of day that you have the food or drink is important, too, so be accurate, and ideally have the diary with you all the time and fill it in as you go. Most important, do not diet! Just eat and drink what you normally do. This is crucial. As much as you might want to jump straight into a new, healthful way of eating, believe it or not, I must stop you. Trust me on this. You, my friend, must understand *why* you are in this mess in the first place. We

learn nothing if we don't know *why*. And isn't that your current mantra, "I don't know why I can't lose weight"? *An accurate and honest diary of what you're eating is the first step!*

Using your calorie counter, work out your total calories for each day and the total for the week. Now you can look at the choices you have been making and decide what needs to change.

Are you skipping breakfast?
Are you eating late?
Are you bingeing at night?
Are your portion sizes on par with those of a 6'6" lumberjack?
Do you eat highly processed, sugary food (chocolate, chips, cake) every day?
Do you avoid green leafy vegetables?
Are you drinking alcohol most nights?
Are you eating out a lot?

The telltale component to all this will be when you add up your calorie intake for the week. If you've been completely honest and not altered your eating habits, it should now be no secret why you are overweight. (By simply cutting out cookies, cakes, candy, and drinking low-fat milk, you'd see an *amazing* difference over several weeks, even if you didn't exercise!)

You need to continue keeping the food diary in your journal, adding up the calories each week, until you reach your goal weight.

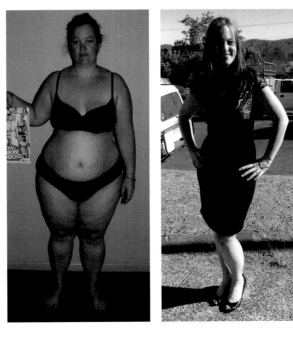

Kristy
Make a plan to change your life!

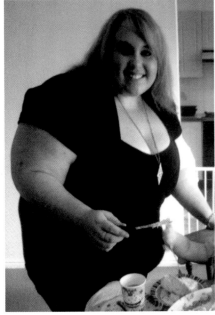

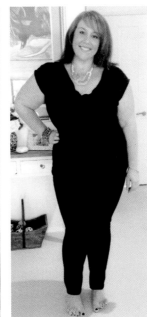

Amy
63 pounds gone for good!

"*Total Body Transformation* changed my life forever. . . . I'm on my way to achieving my lifelong goals."

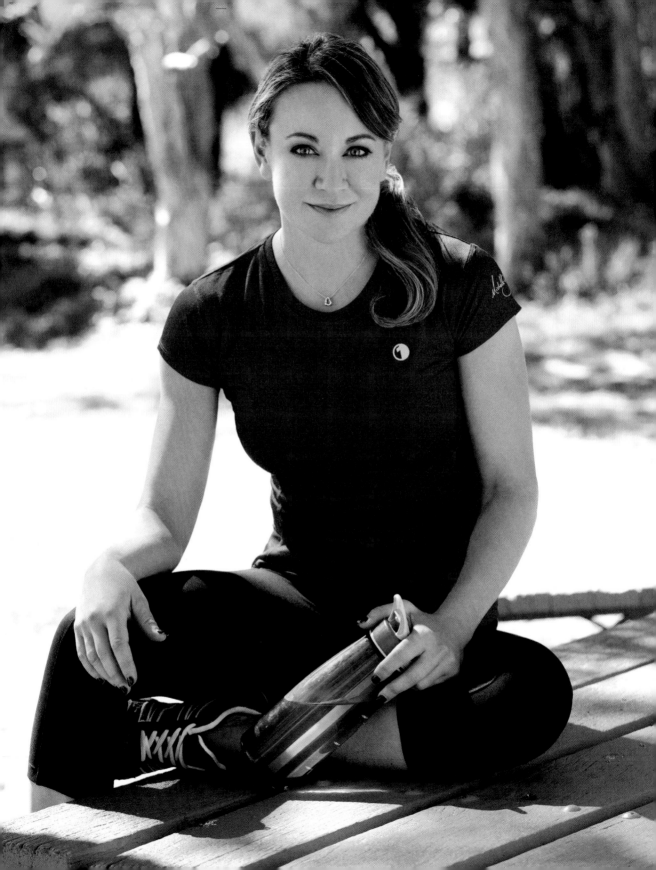

5
do the math

"quantify your weight loss goals to add quality to your life!"

If you're serious about changing your body, you simply cannot be haphazard in your approach to better health and fitness. Fortunately, we have at our disposal the tools to help us determine our ideal body composition, the caloric density of the food we eat, the caloric expenditure of various exercises, and even our basal metabolic rate (I explain this on page 38). While none of these formulas are 100 percent foolproof, they are invaluable for their ability to provide us with guidelines that make getting to our goals a whole lot easier than if we didn't have them.

body mass index

Body mass index (BMI) is a widely used indicator to classify an individual's weight status.

It's essentially a measurement tool that compares your height to your weight to determine whether you are overweight, underweight, or at a healthy weight for your height. It's probably not the best indicator of health risk (your waist measurement is better—see page 36), but it's a pretty useful tool to work out your weight loss goal.

Your BMI is calculated by dividing your weight by your height in inches squared and multiplying that number by 703. So if you're 5'5" tall (65 inches) and weigh 150 pounds, your BMI will be:

$$150 \div (65 \times 65) \times 703 = {\sim}25$$

If you don't have a calculator, use the table on page 39 or the BMI calculator on my website, www.michellebridges.com.

Here's how the classifications look:

- Less than 18: very underweight, you may be malnourished
- Less than 20: slightly underweight, a good meal wouldn't do any harm
- 20 to 25: a healthy weight
- 26 to 30: overweight—time to get moving
- Over 30: obese—the party's over, major lifestyle changes coming your way
- Over 35: severely obese—you must act now to get your life back
- Over 40: morbidly obese—your weight is profoundly affecting the number of years you'll be on the planet complaining about it

Remember that these ratings apply to young and middle-aged adults. They aren't designed for the elderly or for children.

Note, too, that as you lose weight your BMI will drop, so you will need to recalculate it every few weeks. Also, BMI ratings don't apply to athletes who carry a lot of muscle— for example, bodybuilders or people who regularly train with weights. Their BMIs will show them to be overweight or even obese!

waist measurement

While the BMI is a useful indicator of whether someone is overweight, research is showing that waist circumference is probably a better risk indicator of America's number one killer—heart disease. And interestingly, fat deposits around the waist seem to be more dangerous for women than for men.

Waist measurement is important because while you want to look good, you want to look good for *longer*. Keep an eye on this

waist measurement (in) and risk of heart disease

				Not at risk					Increased risk				Substantially increased risk							
30	31	32	33	34	35	36	37	38	39	40	41	42	43	44	45	46	47	48	49	50

MEN

WOMEN

25	26	27	28	29	30	31	32	33	34	35	36	37	38	39	40	41	42	43	44	45
			Not at risk						Increased risk				Substantially increased risk							

measurement and make sure you stay in the safe zone.

calories in, calories out

Okay. You know your goal weight, and you've planned the number of pounds you want to drop each week. Now we get down to the nitty-gritty. Physically, your ability to gain or lose weight is determined by how many calories you eat compared with how many calories you burn. Eat more than you burn, and you get fat. Burn more than you eat, and you get thin. It's that simple. Sure, there are lots of other determining microfactors, but if you're in the market for some serious weight loss, that's all you need to know.

What really leaps out at me when looking at calorie expenditure and exercise is just *how much* you have to do to burn off the calories you've taken on with the odd eating misdemeanor. For example, next time you enjoy just one beer and some potato chips (a 12-oz glass of beer is around 150 calories and a 3½-oz bag of chips is around 500 calories), you can look forward to 1 hour and 10 minutes of full-bore, gut-wrenching cycling to get rid of them! Craving a cappuccino (100 calories) and an extra-large blueberry muffin (500 calories)? Prepare yourself for a 60-minute non-stop jog!

On the face of it, this doesn't seem all that bad, but wash down a croissant or its equivalent with two or more cappuccinos every day of your working week, plus any other crap you might have in your diet, and it's easy to see why you are putting on weight. Add to this, little or no exercise and you *will* be going up a clothing size each year, no doubt about it.

A daily snack like this in the morning or afternoon will give you a calorie load of more than 3,000 calories in just one week—that's nearly *two days'* worth of calories you've just tacked onto your weekly allowance! That equates to a gross weight gain of around 5 pounds a month, which is nearly *50 pounds a year*! Any lightbulbs coming on out there?

Since I've got you on the ropes, let me ruin your day even further with some more examples of the calories in–calories out equation as it applies to a working girl or boy in everyday life (see next page).

The number of calories you can burn off on a walk or run varies from person to person, but I think you get what I'm saying here. One way or another, everything you put into your body will be either converted into energy to fuel movement or converted to your butt size. *This is why people making poor food choices stay overweight even though they are training hard*. They fall for what I call the reward syndrome: "I trained this morning, so I can eat this muffin." I talk more about this on page 57.

Keep in mind that overweight people will generally burn more calories than smaller people, because the more out of shape you are, the harder your heart must work, and the higher your heart rate, the more calories you smash up. However, overweight and unfit individuals generally can't exercise with the same intensity as fitter, thinner people because they have to stop for frequent rests during the same period, which will reduce their overall calorie expenditure.

When you've got a basic understanding of the calorie content of the foods in your life and what it takes to get rid of them, you are better equipped to organize yourself into a calorie-deficit lifestyle. This is why I want you to continue your food diary until you reach your goal weight.

Working out how many calories we eat is the easy bit—we can just look them up in a calorie counter. Working out how many calories we burn each day is a little trickier. We first need to work out our basal metabolic rate (the calories we burn just being alive) and then add any calories we burn through exercise/training.

basal metabolic rate (bmr)

Our BMR describes the calories used to keep our body functioning every day—our lungs full of air, our heart beating, our digestive system going, and so on. We burn these calories when we are literally just sitting around, sleeping, or even flat out in a coma. Our BMR is influenced by a number of factors, including our gender, our age, the amount of muscle we carry, and whether we live in a hot or a cold climate, to name just a few.

The equations on page 40 allow you to calculate your BMR. If you haven't already done so, go and grab a calculator and work out your BMR right now, then write the result in your journal. Or if you prefer, go to my website (www.michellebridges.com) and use the BMR calculator there.

1 glass champagne = 90 cals // Power walk 1.25 miles = 90 cals
1 large chocolate muffin = 500 cals // Jog 4 miles at medium pace = 500 cals
1 chocolate-chip cookie= 90 cals // Run up 15 flights of stairs = 90 cals

BMI body mass index

WEIGHT ▼	4'10"	4'11"	5'0"	5'1"	5'2"	5'3"	5'4"	5'5"	5'6"	5'7"	5'8"	5'9"	5'10"	5'11"	6'0"	6'1"	6'2"	6'3"
100	21	20	20	19	18	18	17	17	16	16	15	15	14	14	14	13	13	13
105	22	21	21	20	19	19	18	18	17	16	16	16	15	15	14	14	14	13
110	23	22	22	21	20	20	19	18	18	17	17	16	16	15	15	15	14	14
115	24	23	23	22	21	20	20	19	19	18	18	17	17	16	16	15	15	14
120	25	24	23	23	22	21	21	20	19	19	18	18	17	17	16	16	15	15
125	26	25	24	24	23	22	22	21	20	20	19	18	18	17	17	17	16	16
130	27	26	25	25	24	23	22	22	21	20	20	19	19	18	18	17	17	16
135	28	27	26	26	25	24	23	23	22	21	21	20	19	19	18	18	17	17
140	29	28	27	27	26	25	24	23	23	22	21	21	20	20	19	19	18	18
145	30	29	28	27	27	26	25	24	23	23	22	21	21	20	20	19	19	18
150	31	30	29	28	27	27	26	25	24	24	23	22	22	21	20	20	19	19
155	32	31	30	29	28	28	27	26	25	24	24	23	22	22	21	20	20	19
160	34	32	31	30	29	28	28	27	26	25	24	24	23	22	22	21	21	20
165	35	33	32	31	30	29	28	28	27	26	25	24	24	23	22	22	21	21
170	36	34	33	32	31	30	29	28	27	27	26	25	24	24	23	22	22	21
175	37	35	34	33	32	31	30	29	28	27	27	26	25	24	24	23	23	22
180	38	36	35	34	33	32	31	30	29	28	27	27	26	25	24	24	23	23
185	39	37	36	35	34	33	32	31	30	29	28	27	27	26	25	24	24	23
190	40	38	37	36	35	34	33	32	31	30	29	28	27	27	26	25	24	24
195	41	39	38	37	36	35	34	33	32	31	30	29	28	27	27	26	25	24
200	42	40	39	38	37	36	34	33	32	31	30	30	29	28	27	26	26	25
205	43	41	40	39	38	36	35	34	33	32	31	30	29	29	28	27	26	26
210	44	43	41	40	38	37	36	35	34	33	32	31	30	29	29	28	27	26
215	45	44	42	41	39	38	37	36	35	34	33	32	31	30	29	28	28	27
220	46	45	43	42	40	39	38	37	36	35	34	33	32	31	30	29	28	28
225	47	46	44	43	41	40	39	38	36	35	34	33	32	31	31	30	29	28
230	48	47	45	44	42	41	40	38	37	36	35	34	33	32	31	30	30	29
235	49	48	46	44	43	42	40	39	38	37	36	35	34	33	32	31	30	29
240	50	49	47	45	44	43	41	40	39	38	37	36	35	34	33	32	31	30
245	51	50	48	46	45	43	42	41	40	38	37	36	35	34	33	32	32	31
250	52	51	49	47	46	44	43	42	40	39	38	37	36	35	34	33	32	31
255	53	52	50	48	47	45	44	43	41	40	39	38	37	36	35	34	33	32
260	54	53	51	49	48	46	45	43	42	41	40	38	37	36	35	34	33	33
265	56	54	52	50	49	47	46	44	43	42	40	39	38	37	36	35	34	33
270	57	55	53	51	49	48	46	45	44	42	41	40	39	38	37	36	35	34

Note: there is a slightly more complicated calculation you can make that takes into account the calories you burn in your daily work, but in my experience, people with weight issues usually lead a sedentary life, or their activity levels can vary greatly, so I tend not to use it. Working from the lowest common denominator—their BMR—means that any extra daily exercise is a bonus for my clients!

exercise expenditure

The next step is working out how many calories you burn up in a training session. If you're not doing any exercise, you'll have nothing to add here, but if you are doing some form of training, your expenditure will vary depending on:

- The type of training
- Your weight
- Your age
- The intensity of your training
- The length of your training

66

+

(6.25 × weight in pounds)

+

(12.7 × height in inches)

−

(6.76 × age in years)

_____

= BMR for males

655

+

(4.35 × weight in pounds)

+

(4.7 × height in inches)

−

(4.68 × age in years)

_____

= BMR for females

The best way to know how many calories you're burning during exercise is by using a heart rate monitor. These display not only your heart rate but also the number of calories you have burned, and they have the added benefit of being *unique* to you. In other words, your heart rate is being calculated by the same equipment every time. Heart rate monitors on gym cardio equipment can vary

calorie expenditure chart for 60 minutes of training

	body weight in lbs						
exercise	**154**	**176**	**198**	**220**	**243**	**265**	**287**
Walk (light)	245	280	315	350	385	420	455
Walk (brisk) 4 mph	280	320	360	400	440	480	520
Slow jog 5 mph	560	640	720	800	880	960	1,040
Jog 6.2 mph	805	920	1,035	1,150	1,265	1,380	1,495
Swim laps	560	640	720	800	880	960	1,040
Cycle 10–12 mph	420	480	540	600	660	720	780
Cycle 12–13.5 mph	700	800	900	1,000	1,100	1,200	1,300
Cycle class (high intensity)	735	840	945	1,050	1,155	1,260	1,365
Group fitness class (high energy)	490	560	630	700	770	840	910
Weights (light)	210	240	270	300	330	360	390
Weights (heavy)	420	480	540	600	660	720	780

from one piece to another, plus they aren't always that accurate. Buy, beg, or borrow a heart rate monitor and strap it on!

Personally, I *always* wear mine when I train. I love knowing how many calories I've chewed up by the end of a training session. In fact, I sometimes use that as part of my training: "Okay, Mishy. You have to expend 600 calories before you can stop, no matter what!"

I also love watching my heart rate while I'm training, as it tells me when I need to take it up a notch or two. Sometimes I use it as a timer when I'm resting and tell myself,

"Okay, Mishy, you can slow down until your heart rate drops to 140, then get back into it!"

If you don't have a heart rate monitor, you can use the Calorie Expenditure Chart above to estimate how many calories you burn during exercise. Figures in the table are really just an estimate but will help you understand the energy in–energy out equation, which is crucial to your weight loss success.

You'll notice that *the heavier you are, the more calories you'll burn,* which is one of the reasons that people carrying a lot of body fat often lose it quickly to start with. But as we know, heavy people are generally pretty unfit

example: client 1

	calories in	BMR	workout	calorie surplus/deficit
Monday	1,290	1,461	323	−494
Tuesday	1,310	1,461	468	−619
Wednesday	1,385	1,461	502	−578
Thursday	1,280	1,461	0	−181
Friday	1,300	1,461	545	−706
Saturday	1,356	1,461	0	−105
Sunday	1,275	1,461	200	−386
total	9,196	10,227	2,038	−3,069

This client is just getting back into shape. She is 5'2" tall and weighs 159 pounds, giving her a body mass index of 29 (see page 35 for an explanation of BMI), putting her into the overweight range. She is thirty-seven years old and works in an office, and her fitness is quite low. Her goal is to lose 30 pounds.

I have set her daily intake at a limit of 1,300 calories and asked her to train six out of seven days, with one day's exercise being a fun bike ride with her family.

She managed to get all her workouts in except for one (Thursday) and did very well cutting her calorie intake. Being 3,069 calories in deficit, she lost only about one pound in one week. Although her goal was to lose 2 pounds in one week, she knew that if she hadn't missed that workout and had amped up her other training sessions, she would have made it. So this was a good lesson. But hey, she's *stoked*! She's got her head sorted out and she feels better than she has in years. Plus, she knows where she's going and she knows she's going to get there. She's taken back control.

The key for her is not to miss her workouts. And right now, two out of the six workouts need to be "gut busters," meaning she will need to tough it out either longer or harder (or both) to burn more calories.

example: client 2

	calories in	BMR	workout	calorie surplus/deficit
Monday	1,780	2,234	1,021	−1,475
Tuesday	1,630	2,234	773	−1,377
Wednesday	1,700	2,234	952	−1,486
Thursday	1,600	2,234	910	−1,544
Friday	1,610	2,234	1,100	−1,724
Saturday	3,500	2,234	898	368
Sunday	1,650	2,234	0	−584
total	13,470	15,638	5,654	7,822

This guy is thirty-five years old, weighs 234 pounds, and is 6'2" tall. His basal metabolic rate works out to be 2,234. His goal is to lose 30 pounds.

We started his daily calorie intake at 1,700 and his training at one hour a day, five times a week. Two sessions were with me and three on his own. I asked him to be more active on day six and to rest on day seven. His treat meal (see page 183) is Saturday night. On Saturday he decided to do an extra workout so that he felt free to indulge, and he also made a conscious effort to increase his daily activity levels—taking the stairs, walking to meetings, and so on.

By the end of the week on paper we had him pegged at just over 2 pounds down. However, due to increased general activity levels (taking the stairs, etc.), the scale showed him as 4 pounds down, and he was thrilled. (Remember, the human body is not like a computer—hormones, stress, and activity levels can throw off your careful calculations, often for the better. The key is to be consistent and stay on course.)

Because we had gone through smart food choices, he did not feel hungry, and although he admitted that he occasionally thought about cheating, he waited for Saturday night, which he thoroughly enjoyed.

and can't keep up the intensity in their training, so their weight loss often slows right down. The trick is to get fit as soon as you can because then you'll get the best of both worlds.

My experience in *The Biggest Loser* house reinforced this. It was not uncommon for some of the contestants to rip up over 1,000 calories in a 50-minute session! They were super-fit close to the end of the show even though they were still overweight, and their newfound fitness, coupled with an increase in their muscle mass, meant that they were incinerating calories in their workouts and stripping body fat like crazy. Way to go!

So your simple weight loss calculation will look like this:

> basal metabolic rate
> + calorie expenditure
> = calories burned
>   for the day

start counting

Okay, now that you know how many calories you're burning, you can figure out if you're in calorie surplus or calorie deficit:

> calories in
> − calories out
> =calorie surplus
>   or calorie deficit

To lose weight, you need to be in *calorie deficit*. In order to lose one pound per week you will need to be in deficit of around 3,500 calories. Go back to your SMART objectives (page 19) and remind yourself how many pounds a week you need to lose to reach your goal.

Now grab your journal and calculate your required weekly calorie deficit. If you need to drop, say, two pounds each week, your calorie deficit needs to be around 7,000 calories. Along with your food diary, you need to keep a daily tally of your calories in and calories out. (See page 232 for a template, or download one from my website.) You absolutely *must* be committed to keeping your records. This is what I expect from all my clients, and I've included a couple of examples here to help you get started (see pages 42–43).

transformation story!

After losing 70 pounds and going from 210 to 140 pounds, I still felt I had weight to lose. I tried more exercise, then I tried to diet, but nothing seemed to work for me. Michelle's exercise program was like having a personal trainer twenty-four hours a day. If I missed a gym class, I could use the gym machines, or even work out in the local park (which I really enjoyed). And I loved having a ready-made menu that took

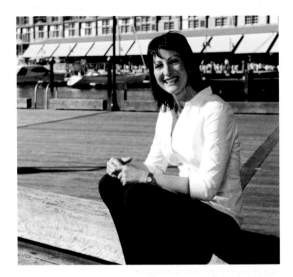

Maureen Crook

the guesswork out of dinner. Not only did I get to my goal weight of 130 pounds, but I now weigh 125! I feel fantastic and am so happy with myself!

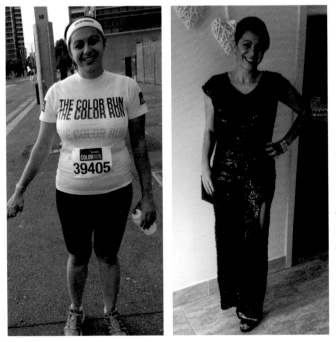

Diala
Be stronger and leaner than you
ever thought possible.

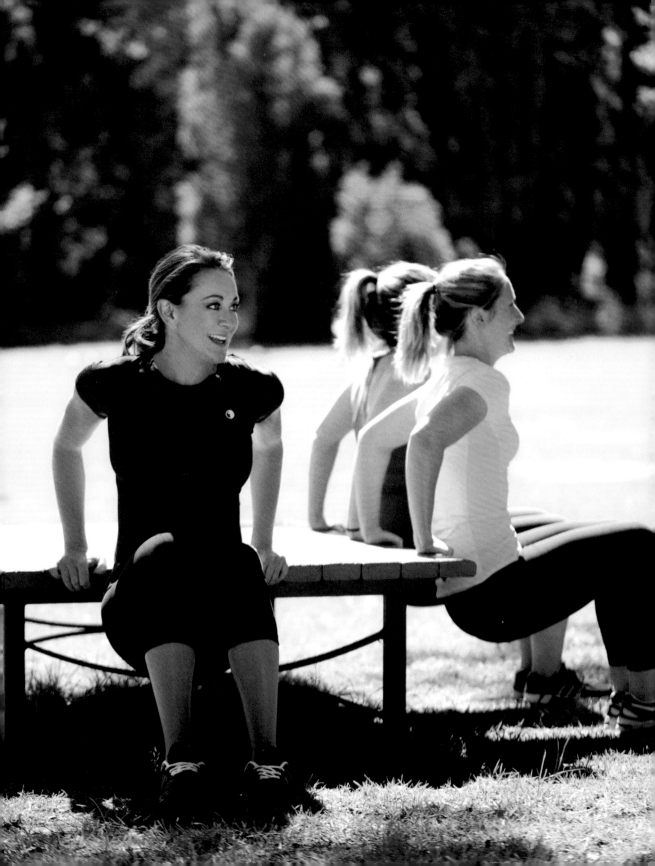

6
debunking the myths

"separate fact from fiction, then get moving!"

Being in the fitness industry for as long as I have has exposed me to lots of useful information and experience, and also to a lot of crap. Let's see if we can clear the decks before we set sail.

myth 1: walking is a great way to get fit and lose weight

Using myself as an example, I know that if I power-walk for 10 minutes on a flat road, I will burn around 20 calories, which is about the calorie content of a raw carrot. By comparison, if I run for 10 minutes on a flat road at about 6 mph, I will burn around 100 calories, which is a 12-ounce skim latte with no sugar.

Now, when the number one excuse for not exercising is that we don't have enough time, I know which exercise routine I would rather devote my 10 minutes to. If you only have 30 minutes to dedicate to exercise, then passive exercise isn't really going to give you the results you are looking for, and frankly I categorize walking the dog or taking a morning walk with a girlfriend for a chat as "passive exercise."

In other words, if you want to lose weight at a reasonable rate, then forget walking because your calorie expenditure just isn't time-efficient. You'd need to walk at a brisk pace for 45 minutes just to burn off the coffee that you'd probably have afterward, in which case the net benefit to your weight loss goals would be *zero*.

"nothing, but nothing, holds back the years like weight training."

There's nothing wrong with going for a walk. In fact, it's one of the best ways to clear your head, get some fresh air, and lift your spirits. But if your goal is to burn off excess body fat and calories, then you'll probably find yourself becoming highly unmotivated, because it's not going to get you the results you're after.

Having said that, we've all got to start somewhere, and walking *is* a great place to start. But allow me to emphasize the word *start*. You must be ready to push your boundaries at every session and never go back. Your plan should be to graduate from walking to power-walking, then timing your power walks and gradually upping the intensity so that you either walk farther or walk the same distance in less time. From there you add some jogging along the way, and so on.

So don't whine to me that nothing is changing for you physically when your formal exercise program continues to be a casual stroll with your girlfriend. This kind of passive exercise is good because you're moving, but it's not what you should be spending a lot of time doing if you're trying to lose weight.

myth 2: low-intensity exercise burns more fat than high-intensity exercise

The argument here is that low-intensity exercise sources almost all of its energy from fat stores, which is true. This little charmer was put out by the equipment manufacturers to encourage more people to cruise around the cardio gear thinking they were burning fat because they were training at 65 percent of their maximum heart rate while flicking through a copy of *Cosmopolitan*. Now, low-intensity exercise *does* chew into body fat, but you need to be there *a lot longer* to burn off a decent number of calories. And let's recall the number one reason for *not* exercising: "I don't have enough time." So it's a no-brainer! Train smarter and harder, then get the hell outta there! High-intensity exercise uses *bucketloads* of energy and hence plenty of fat. Plus, the harder you train, the fitter you get; the fitter you get, the harder you can train and the more calories you can expend.

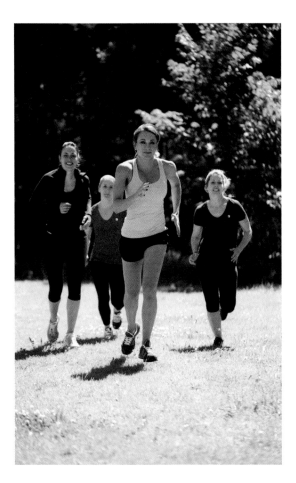

headed and can't train as hard as you'd like, then don't blow off the workout—eat a light snack half an hour beforehand. A piece of fruit is usually the best thing. Personally, I love training before breakfast.

myth 4: you shouldn't train with weights every day

Can anybody tell me why not? Sure, you need to give your body time to recover from a hard weight-training session (note the word *hard*), but you can still train with weights every day if you are training specific parts of the body in each session. For example: legs on Monday, chest and biceps on Tuesday, back and triceps on Wednesday, and so on.

I get quizzed a lot about the risk of "overtraining," but I have to be honest with you on this one. Olympians, professional athletes, yes, they can be exposed to overtraining. But the average overweight American? Ah . . . not many overtrainers there. Anyone asking me about overtraining is usually looking for an excuse *not* to train.

If you're in a gym, the idea is to use a variety of workouts to keep up the interest level, or if you have a favorite, vary the intensity so you can do it day after day. (I show you how to set up your own workouts with minimal

myth 3: never train on an empty stomach

Well, this one is the source of plenty of debate. When you haven't eaten for a while, such as first thing in the morning, your body is glycogen-depleted and you are more likely to use stored fat as an energy source.

If, though, you find you become light-equipment in Chapter 8.) The key is to stick to your schedule no matter what. As soon as you miss a training session, it becomes easier to blow off the next one. Before you know it, three months have gone by and you've done nothing.

You'll need to be tough and work around injuries. If you've got blisters, bandage them up and keep going. If you've pulled a muscle in your shoulder, train your lower body, and train it harder. Just *do not stop*.

myth 5: pilates, yoga, and stretch classes are great for weight loss

Okay, let me lay this on you. Pilates and stretch classes are fantastic for posture, strength, flexibility, and mind-body connection. But for weight loss? *Shithouse*. The heart rate simply isn't elevated enough to burn calories at any significant rate. If you want to slip in a Pilates class to help with core strength, or a yoga session to improve your flexibility and quiet your mind, that's fine, but if you want to lose weight, you're barking up the wrong tree pose.

myth 6: you can spot-reduce fat

I'm sick of answering this one. No, you can't. End of story. Next question?

myth 7: women get big if they train with weights

Um, last time I checked, us chicks were loaded up with a little thing called estrogen, which makes it tough to build muscle mass. For that you need testosterone. We can all change the shape of our bodies for the better with resistance training, which means that your muscles will become more defined, toned, and shapely. I continually get women who come to me overjoyed with their physiques after I've put them on a weight program. Nothing, but nothing, holds back the years like weight training.

There is so much information out there now that tells us about the benefits of weight training for both men and women that you'd have to be nuts not to do it. Eating and drinking too much garbage will make you big! Training with weights won't! Unless of course your personal trainer's called Wolfgang von Fraudenspanker and he's wearing a 1972 East German Olympic tracksuit. Please!

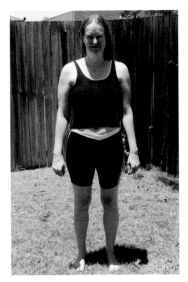
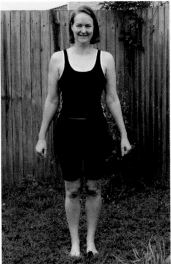

Sarah and Matt
Together Matt and Sarah have lost
70 pounds!

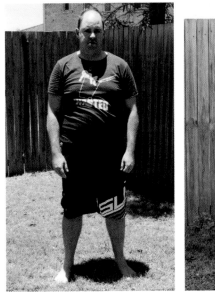
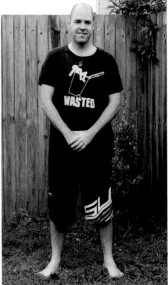

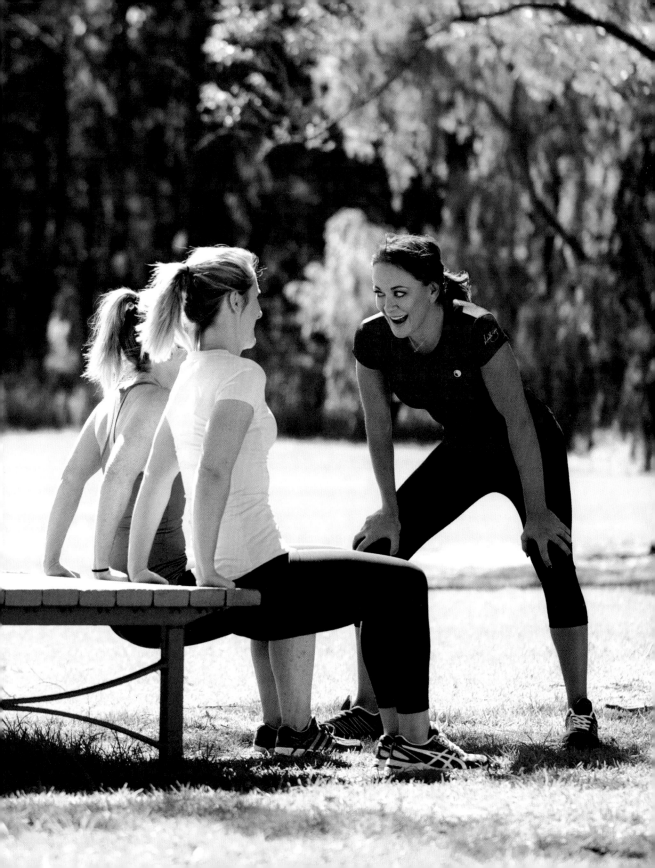

7
tips, tricks, and pitfalls

"we all need a cheat sheet sometimes."

Okay, you're passionately committed to becoming a leaner, fitter you, and you've worked out how to track your progress by measuring calories in versus calories out. Now you are going to *exercise*. That's right. You will be an exerciser, forever. Not just until you fit into that dress, or until your birthday, or till you look great so you can dump your boyfriend while looking hot. No. You are an exerciser. Period.

Exercise is the fountain of youth. Research shows that it not only acts as a preventative, relieving you of the stresses and anxieties that can bring about illness, but also has amazing curative properties. Researchers at Duke University, for example, studied people suffering from depression for four months and found that 60 percent of the participants

who exercised for just 30 minutes three times a week overcame their depression without antidepressant medication.

Not only does exercise make you stronger, fitter, and lighter, but you get to live a more productive and active life *for longer*. Not because you are on a cocktail of drugs and have to sit at your window with a blanket over your lap and watch the world go by until you die. You get to be independent, empowered, healthy, and fit, and probably end up kicking the bucket in a skiing accident at the age of ninety-three! And still a size 8!

Clearly, exercise does so much more than help you lose weight. It's actually unnatural for us *not* to exercise, and we are seeing the results of this with surging levels of obesity, mental illness, diabetes, heart disease, and other illnesses that have evolved and multiplied as a result of our sedentary lifestyles.

we are designed to move!

If you look at the human body, it's designed to move. We have multiple movable joints that allow us to do so much more than sit on a couch.

Yet here is an example of an everyday person's daily activity schedule:

1. Wake up
2. Sit down to eat breakfast (maybe)
3. Get in car and drive to work
4. Get in elevator to get to office
5. Sit at desk
6. Eat lunch at desk
7. Get in elevator to get back to car
8. Get home and sit down to dinner
9. Sit in front of TV
10. Get into bed

Next day—press repeat.

For a lot of us, this is a snapshot of our everyday lives, and it doesn't even take into account the health implications and weight issues that go with such a zero-movement lifestyle.

When it comes to our bodies, the old "use it or lose it" mantra goes for everything—bones, muscles, heart, lungs, and brain. This fact is backed up by a multitude of research, but my favorite study was carried out by a man named K. N. Pavlou and his team in 1985. He got two groups of mildly overweight men and put them both on a rapid weight loss diet for eight weeks. He also got one of the groups doing aerobic exercise three times a week. The exercising group lost 26 pounds in total, and the non-exercising group lost 20 pounds. Not much difference, I hear you say. Except that of the 26 pounds lost by the exercising group, a full 95 percent of it was fat loss! This compares to only 64 percent fat loss by the non-exercisers. The exercisers also looked better and were better equipped to keep losing weight because their metabolisms had elevated.

So when you're stripping weight off, hang on to the muscle, because you're gonna need it!

where to start

You are about to send your body into a state of shock. If you have never exercised, or even if you're a lapsed exerciser, your body is about to get the biggest wake-up call it's had in years. But unlike your old self, who would punish your body by eating crap and being inactive, you're going to dish out tough love by *working* your body and working it hard.

Get the distinction: on the face of it, your old self would have been "spoiling" your body by feeding it sugary garbage and deep-fried whatever, but in fact you were punishing it because you hated it. The term *spoiling* is actually spot-on, because that's literally what you were doing—ruining it. Now, though, you love your body. You embrace, accept, and revere it, and you do that by taking it to hell and back!

When I train people for the first time I show them no mercy, and although their minds quickly buckle and fall apart, their bodies don't. So when you're telling yourself, "I can't do this, it's too hard," that's not your body talking. It's your mind. And it's your mind that has gotten your body where it is today.

get a checkup

Before you start exercising, you'll need to see your doctor for a checkup. Some people with certain illnesses or who are taking particular medications may have difficulty losing weight easily. They will need to approach my weight loss program under their practitioner's supervision. Whatever your circumstances, tell your doctor that you're leaving this overweight, unhealthy body right there in the waiting room and that you will need his or her support. This journey is best taken with as much help as you can get, so if there's a lot of negative talk around, I recommend you get rid of Dr. Do-Little and find a practitioner who's on the same page.

I see many people start off with the best of intentions but then get sick a couple of weeks in. After that, the comeback is even harder than the first session and it all quickly falls apart. That's when I hear, "Oh, I tried going to the gym but it didn't work for me," usually around the barbecue (another pork sausage, anyone? Come on, they're only seven billion calories . . .).

People who haven't exercised in fifteen years will often get sick after the first few workouts because their bodies are so busy trying to repair themselves that their immune systems are compromised. You've got to understand that your body is going to be *screaming* for nutrients and rest to help it recover when you get started on your exercise program.

get plenty of rest

Go to bed half an hour earlier, and if you're a poor sleeper (which you may well be if you're overweight) take steps to improve your sleep quality. These steps can include:

- **No stimulants after midday.** This includes caffeine, soft drinks, and chocolate—the last two help you to gain weight, so they should be ditched anyway. Oh, and did I mention cigarettes? Kick those suckers to the curb.
- **Invest in a good bed.** If you're wrestling with your partner over mattress space all night, then get yourself a bigger one (bigger bed, that is—not a bigger partner).
- **Make sure your bedroom is dark.** If your curtains or blinds let light through, replace them with ones that don't.
- **Try using lavender oil with a fragrance oil warmer in the bedroom.** Lavender is known for its calming and soothing properties. (Don't forget to blow out the tealight candle before you go to sleep.)
- **Keep all electronics out of the bedroom.** No TVs or computers.

drink lots of water

Most of us just don't drink enough water. While training, you should be aiming for at least 64 ounces a day (see "How Much Water?" on page 11 to calculate your ideal water goal). Many people actually confuse thirst with hunger. If you think you're hungry long before you're due for your next meal, try drinking a large glass of water—it will often dampen hunger pangs. Everything functions better when you are well hydrated, and if you've waited till you're thirsty, you've waited too long. Your pee will let you know if you are hydrated or not. Have no fear if it's clear. It's all wrong if there's a strong smell!

eat regularly and well

Eat well (see "Let's Get Cooking!") and take simple supplements (a multivitamin-mineral combo plus vitamin C). Avoid megavitamins—you don't need massive doses. Supplements should be taken with or immediately before or after food, as this helps with their absorption.

A low-calorie diet and especially one low in fat can disrupt the balance of cholesterol and bile salts in your body, leading to the formation of gallstones. Bile is stored in the gallbladder until it's needed for metabolizing fats. If it stays there too long—because there's no fat to break down—little "stones" develop. Eating regularly and including some

"aerobic activity is your number one weight loss weapon."

good fats in your diet will keep the gallbladder working and releasing bile into your digestive system. But before you reach for that chocolate bar, consider that a couple of slices of Arnold Health Nut bread will provide 4 grams of fat, none of which are saturated, plus 10 grams of protein. Caffeine and small quantities of monounsaturated fats such as flaxseed oil, sesame oil, or olive oil will help to reduce the risks.

Even without dieting, if you are overweight you already have an increased risk of developing gallstones. Studies have shown that a woman with a BMI of 30 or more has double the risk of gallstones than a woman with a BMI of less than 25. Women are more likely to form gallstones than men, particularly if there's a history of gallstones in your family. I know, girls—just add it to periods and uncomfortable heels.

Recent studies at Flinders University in South Australia have shown that weight loss candidates who lose more than 1.7 percent of their body weight per week for extended periods are up to ten times more likely to develop gallstones, so if you experience rapidly increasing pain in your right upper abdomen that lasts between 30 minutes and a couple

of hours, or pain between your shoulder blades or under your right shoulder, please see your doctor.

beware the reward syndrome

I find a lot of people who embark on an exercise program can fall into this trap: "I trained today, therefore I can eat XYZ." I can't begin to tell you the number of people I've seen year after year coming to the gyms I work in, endlessly doing the classes and programs prescribed by their personal trainers, but for whom nothing has changed weightwise. And it's not just gym goers—I see the same thing happening with people who are exercising outdoors, jogging, or whatever. I even see it with fitness professionals.

Then they corner me at a social gathering, with a glass of beer in one hand, a piece of pie in the other, and proceed to quiz me about why they can't lose the weight! What they don't understand is that when it comes to weight loss, it's about everything you put in your mouth, not just food but alcohol and soft drinks, too. With the reward syndrome, you'll take two steps forward, then two (or

Don't Stop, Louise!

My girlfriend Louise is built like a greyhound and is a perfect candidate for long-distance running, but unfortunately had never been particularly fit or confident in her physical ability.

An academic, she'd never really done much running, but one day she decided she wanted to go out for a bit of a jog with me. We had planned to run about 3 miles, but we were only about halfway into the first mile when she said she'd have to stop for a breather.

I said quietly, "Why don't we just slow down a bit? We won't stop and walk, but we'll just do a slow shuffle, enough to catch our breath. In fact, it doesn't even matter if we shuffle slower than we could walk."

Although she agreed, I could see that she wasn't happy about the idea. She definitely would have preferred to stop and walk. As we shuffled along, I explained to her that we were far better taking the pressure off and slowing down to a very controlled shuffle than walking. This is because once you stop, it's very hard to start again.

I also reminded her that she was not dying. She was breathing, her heart was beating, she was still moving, and she was not about to expire. She was too concerned with how uncomfortable she was feeling to acknowledge that the puffing and panting, the tightening muscles, the sweating, and the elevated heart rate were signs that her body was working perfectly—exactly as it should do under those circumstances.

"A lot of this is in your head, Lou," I assured her. "Sure, it's a bit uncomfortable, but you're okay. There's nothing to be afraid of. Your body's working just fine."

We ended up running the remaining 2+ miles without stopping, and she was terrific! Exhausted, but terrific! Lou tells me now that this was a turning point for her. "Mishy, I just wanted to stop, but when you said I could take the pressure off and just shuffle, it felt less threatening. And even though I *thought* I couldn't run that far, somehow I did. When you reminded me that I wasn't dying and that a lot of it was in my head, that made total sense to me."

She went on to explain that she never thought that she could be athletic and sporty because she wasn't fit and just "no good" at physical training. She explained that at a young age she'd convinced herself she was the academic type, not the sporty type. "I was pigeonholed, Mishy!" she exclaimed.

What a great result! Louise now actually enjoys her running—something that she never dreamed she would be able to do, and mostly because she had convinced herself that she couldn't. She is now off to Norway to run a half marathon later in the year. Go, Louise!

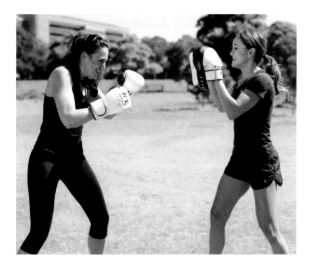

find a training buddy

A training buddy can really help you stay focused—it doesn't matter if your buddy is not as charged up as you. Share your goals with each other so that you stay honest, and when one of you tries to back out of a session, the other can say, "Hang on! You said you wanted to be in a bikini by summer!"

even three) steps backward, which can be really disheartening, especially when you think of all those hours of hard training that you've done. No doubt you'll be fitter, but a size 8 you won't be.

do more informal exercise

If you go to the gym three times a week, on the face of it that sounds pretty good. But 3 out of 112 waking hours is a drop in the ocean if you are sitting on your butt for the rest of the time. If formal exercise is training in the gym, jogging, or playing sports, then informal exercise is taking the stairs, walking to work, bike riding on the weekend, or working hard in the garden. Formal exercise + informal exercise = results!

aerobic training

There are three main forms of exercise: aerobic exercise (also called cardio training), strength training (aka weight training), and flexibility training. Know this: if you want to make a positive impact on your health and well-being, *any* one of these types of exercise will help you. But if you want to lose weight, you need to structure your exercise regime around the exercise that will make you lose weight *fast*. Typically, aerobic exercise (also referred to as cardio training, as it lifts your heart rate) includes jogging, cycling, rowing, and group fitness classes such as step or indoor cycling. In fact, it's pretty much any activity that gets you huffing and puffing. When you're training aerobically, you source energy not only from oxygen but also from carbohydrates and, you guessed it, fat. So aerobic activity is your *number one weight loss weapon*, which is why I recommend you get

"the harder your heart is pumping, the more energy (and calories) you're burning."

yourself a heart rate monitor. This is your *fat-burning meter,* and it also shows your calorie expenditure. The harder your heart is pumping, the more energy (and calories) you're burning.

"So why can't I just go for a run every day to lose the weight?" I hear you ask. Good question. Here are the answers:

- If you've bought this book, there's a fair chance you're not someone who has the technique or stamina to get the results you want from running, especially if you are planning to drop more than 20 pounds. (Though by the time you finish my workout program you will be a mean machine!)
- The structure of a workout program keeps you focused and honest. You are more likely to blow off a training session if you think it's just a couple of laps around the block.
- The strength component (weights) of your training will transform your metabolism from a two-stroke engine to a V8—you'll trash calories *way* faster, and that's what you're here for.

- Having a range of fun and challenging exercises sparks your motivation and interest. (If you're bored, it's pretty easy to roll over and press the snooze button.)
- Once your body becomes accustomed to one kind of aerobic exercise (in this case, running), your calorie burning will plateau and you won't be able to drop as much weight.
- My training program teaches you to be a *savvy exerciser* who can adapt your exercise to work around injuries and changed circumstances—these are skills you will have *for the rest of your life.*

As we've seen, intensity in exercise is *crucial* to getting the results you want, and knowing your heart rate is a way of measuring how intensely you are exercising. You can also use it to push yourself to your desired intensity level. It's a bit like having a training partner or a mean cow like me yelling at you! Your workouts become more scientific, and you can really keep a close eye on *exactly* what's going on with your body while you're training: "Am I burning fat right now? How many calories have I nuked?"

calculating your MHR

The heart rates you'll be aiming for in your workouts are usually expressed as a percentage of your maximum heart rate (MHR).

There are several ways to calculate your MHR, the most common way being to subtract your age from 220—although this doesn't accurately apply to children, the elderly, or the very fit; it's really only a guide.

Your heart rate determines the energy sources your body uses, so broadly speaking you're burning fat almost exclusively (but not much of it) at around 65 percent of your MHR, and a much bigger combo of fat, carbs (in the form of glycogen), and oxygen at around 85 percent of your MHR. For example, if you're thirty years old your MHR is 190, so 65 percent of that is 124 beats per minute and 85 percent is 162 bpm.

interval training

Interval training is where you train at, say, 65–70 percent of your MHR but then periodically ramp it up to, say, 85 percent for a short burst. In practical terms, it's like jogging around a football field but then breaking into a sprint across each end. This kind of exercise really improves your fitness and is one of my faves.

Recent studies at the University of New South Wales have shown just how effective interval training really is, partly because it releases catecholamines that help singe the fat from your backside. From an exerciser's point of view, if you're told that you have to go all out for 30 seconds and then you'll get 30 seconds' rest, you're more likely to rise to the occasion. By contrast, if you are told to go at the same intensity for a full hour, you'd probably balk at the proposition and get a new trainer.

circuit training

Most of my clients follow training programs that they can do without me, so when it's time to train *with* me I usually do some sort of crazy circuit training that's new and interesting for them.

A circuit is a series of "stations" where you exercise for a specified time or perform a specified number of repetitions of an exercise. These can be strength-based stations, cardio-based stations, a mix of the two, all upper body, all lower body, or both. You can time how long it takes you to get through all of the stations and then try to beat your time, or you can sprint four lengths of the room before you go to the next station. The combinations are bound only by your imagination and repertoire of exercises. Sometimes when I train with my *Biggest Loser* co-star, Shannan Ponton, we take turns making up the next exercise, so we never really know what the session will look like till it's over and we're both destroyed. It's perverse, I know, but we're freaks.

plyometrics

Plyometric exercises (or plyos, as I like to call them) are used by sports people to build explosive strength and stamina. They feature a lot of jumping, bounding, throwing, and pushing. They work well with cardiovascular and weight training, as they tend to help "spike" your heart rate, and they get you very, very fit. These exercises are *hard*, and I usually include them in intermediate rather than beginners' programs, so there are only a couple in your workouts.

group fitness classes

Group fitness is sweeping the planet because, unlike the old days, when aerobics all got a bit complicated, modern classes have better-trained instructors and a wider range of class options. Apart from being fun, they have other benefits:

- You don't have to think about what you're going to do—simply turn up and let your instructor do the thinking for you.
- They are held at specific times, ensuring that you actually *do* your training.
- They are safe because there is always an instructor watching what you're doing.
- There is an enormous range of classes. Apart from the conventional aerobics classes that began back in the eighties, there are now pre-choreographed classes that instructors learn. These are well researched, less complex, and easier to participate in, particularly if you've never ventured into a group fitness class before.
- You don't need to buy any gear.

There are loads of classes out there, such as those by Les Mills International. I've been involved with them for over a decade and particularly like their BodyPump (weights), BodyBalance (passive), and BodyAttack (cardio) classes.

weight training

Strength training, weight training, or resistance training—whatever you want to call it—is generally not included in weight loss programs because it sources carbohydrates for energy rather than fats. These carbohydrates have been converted into glycogen (a type of sugar), which is stored in your muscles and in your liver. Unused carbohydrates are stored on your butt.

However, strength training is invaluable in a weight loss program if it is done properly, that is, with sufficient speed and intensity to get your heart rate up. I get sick of seeing guys with big chests and skinny legs meander through their weight workouts and then complain to their friends about the size of their beer gut. Show me a weight trainer who trains hard with urgency and intensity and I'll show you one lean rock star!

Training with weights has its own language. Exercises are usually performed in "sets," with each set made up of a prescribed number of repetitions or "reps." For example, your workout may include three sets of leg presses, with each set consisting of 12 reps.

Because I know the value of strength training for weight loss, you'll notice that many of the workouts in this book include weights. Importantly, all of the weight exercises are set out in the form of "super sets," where you perform two sets of different exercises with-

main muscle groups

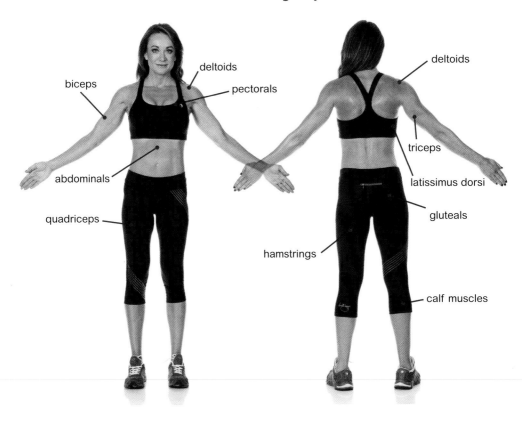

biceps
deltoids
pectorals
abdominals
quadriceps

deltoids
triceps
latissimus dorsi
gluteals
hamstrings
calf muscles

weight loss? Unless you're in a crazy Iyengar yoga class, *forget it*.

One of my clients was only doing this type of training and couldn't figure out why her butt was not getting any smaller. Couple that with her use of the reward syndrome ("I have trained today, so therefore I can have this half bottle of wine") and she was going backward. I took out four of the five Pilates sessions she was doing a week (she kept one), replaced them with cardio, strength, indoor cycling, and a step class, and cleaned out her diet, and she dropped 6 pounds in the first week! Yee-ha!

out a rest in between. This will get your heart rate up, improve your strength and endurance, and *trash* fat cells.

flexibility training

Flexibility training, or passive exercise, includes stretch classes, Pilates, yoga, and the like. Passive exercise improves core strength, relaxation, and flexibility, which is good for everyone (especially as we get older), but for

richard

I met Richard, one of my long-term personal training clients, on a treadmill. I was running on mine, and he was trying to walk on his, though the treadmill kept stalling. Sensing his frustration, I stopped and offered some help, which he gladly accepted. After a quick chat I learned that this was his second session at the gym. He'd joined a week before and was on a "mission" to lose weight. "I'd love to be able to run like you. Maybe in another lifetime!" was his throwaway line.

"Well, that attitude will get you nowhere!" I replied. "I could have you running the City to Surf [a road race in Sydney, Australia] if you really wanted to; you just have to want it enough."

I guess it was a bit cruel of me to throw down the gauntlet like that; I mean, what else could he say but yes? So we organized to start training the following week. In the meantime, his homework was to complete a 7-Day Food Diary (while not dieting) and go to the doctor for a checkup. A week later we did the numbers, and the stats went like this:

Age: 39 years, male

Weight: 268 pounds

Height: 6'2"

Waist measurement: 47 inches

Weight classification: morbidly obese

BMR: 2,363

Blood pressure: 145/87 (dangerously high)

Then he showed me his diary. I won't list the whole thing, just a weekday and a Saturday, but you'll get the idea:

Tuesday			Calories
	7 a.m.	1 large latte with whole milk and 2 sugars	250
	9 a.m.	Whole-wheat roll with 3 fried eggs and ketchup	470
	11 a.m.	1 large latte with whole milk and 2 sugars	250
	1:30 p.m.	Grilled fish, salad, small buttered roll, 2 glasses wine	710
	5 p.m.	1 chocolate bar	200
	5:30 p.m.	1 large latte with whole milk and 2 sugars	250
	8:30 p.m.	1 large bowl of vegetable soup	190
		1 large roll with butter	280
		Veal with pasta	400
		2 glasses red wine	200
		2 small scoops gelato	200
Total			3,400

Saturday			Calories
	8:30 a.m.	1 large latte with whole milk and 2 sugars	250
	10 a.m.	2 poached eggs	146
		1 slice toast with butter	200
		3 slices bacon	390
		Tomato	20
		1 large latte with whole milk and 2 sugars	250
	2 p.m.	1 bag chips (2 oz)	260
		2 sausages in rolls	300
		6 beers	900
	7:30 p.m.	Large steak	300
		Salad	30
		Half slice chocolate cake	170
		3 glasses red wine	300
Total			3,516

Richard's total calories for the week were a whopping 26,000! I was blown away. How was this man still functioning? How come he wasn't suffering some chronic ailment, like *death*? He was scarfing down vast quantities of calorie-dense foods, and all at the wrong times. And he'd only had one day that week without alcohol. No wonder he felt tired a lot and often had headaches and indigestion.

I rewrote his nutrition plan and put him on 1,800–1,900 calories per day with a goal weight of 202 pounds by the time the 8.7-mile City to Surf run came up. That meant he had five months to drop 66 pounds—tight, but doable.

Richard was scared, excited, and pumped all at the same time. Perfect! He trained with me twice a week and did four sessions on his own, two of which were group fitness classes (indoor cycling and weight training). The other two sessions were a mix of weights and cardio. We set up his workout plan so it fit in with his busy schedule and he trained early mornings or lunchtimes, as he often had to stay at work late.

We went through menus and I showed him how to order well while eating out. I also set up some non-negotiable rules, including five alcohol-free days per week, never going back for seconds, and breakfast every day. As for the rest of his nutrition, we gradually got him to a place where he was organized, feeling full, and sticking to the plan. His doctor also prescribed medium-strength hypertension medication for his blood pressure.

At his first weigh-in (a week after he'd started) he'd lost an amazing 12.8 pounds, and he was *stoked*! After one month he was down to 243 pounds, and his hypertension medication was reduced to a low dosage. The second month was a little slower in the weight loss stakes, but he was still losing weight *and* getting fitter. He even joined the gym's running club and found he was easily keeping up at beginner level. By the end of the third month he weighed in at 215 pounds. He looked terrific and was running for 5 miles nonstop! His next goal was the City to Surf; he had two months to train, and he trained *hard*. He was now off his blood pressure medication (his blood pressure clocked in at a healthy 125/75). Inspired by his success, Richard's wife had also started losing weight and exercising, too—a delight for both of them.

Richard ran the City to Surf nonstop, in just 1 hour 48 minutes—an incredible result. I was there to meet him at the finish line. He cried, I cried—soppy, I know, but this man had reinvented himself in just *twenty weeks*! Today Richard weighs 198 pounds and trains five to six days a week. He loves his life and he's looking forward to being a dad.

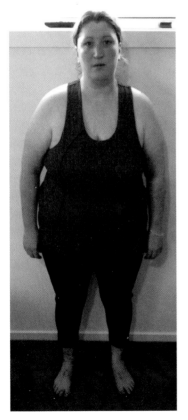 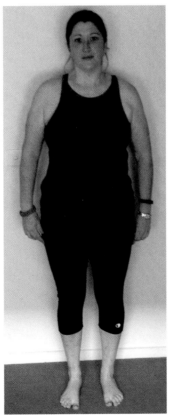

Michaela
101 pounds gone forever!

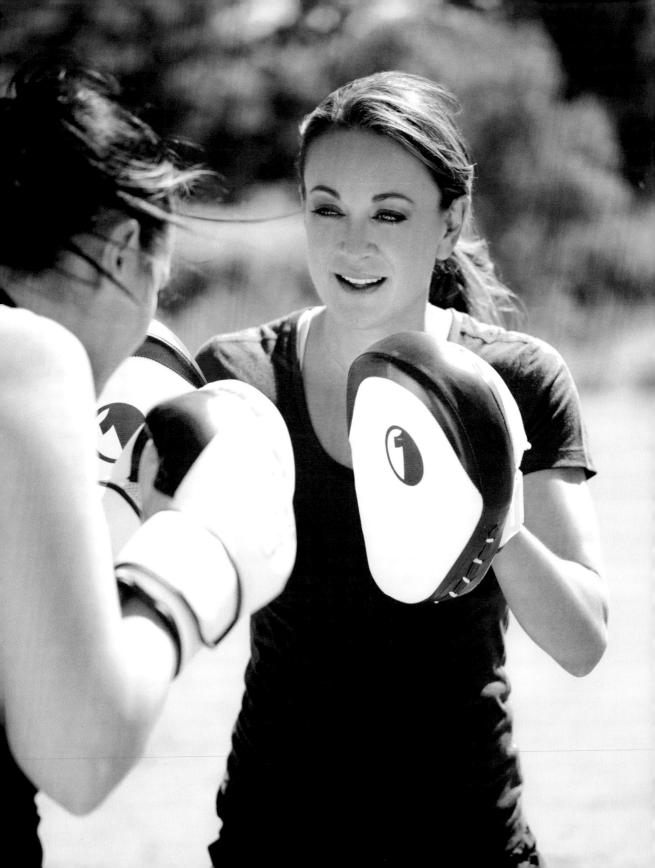

let's train!

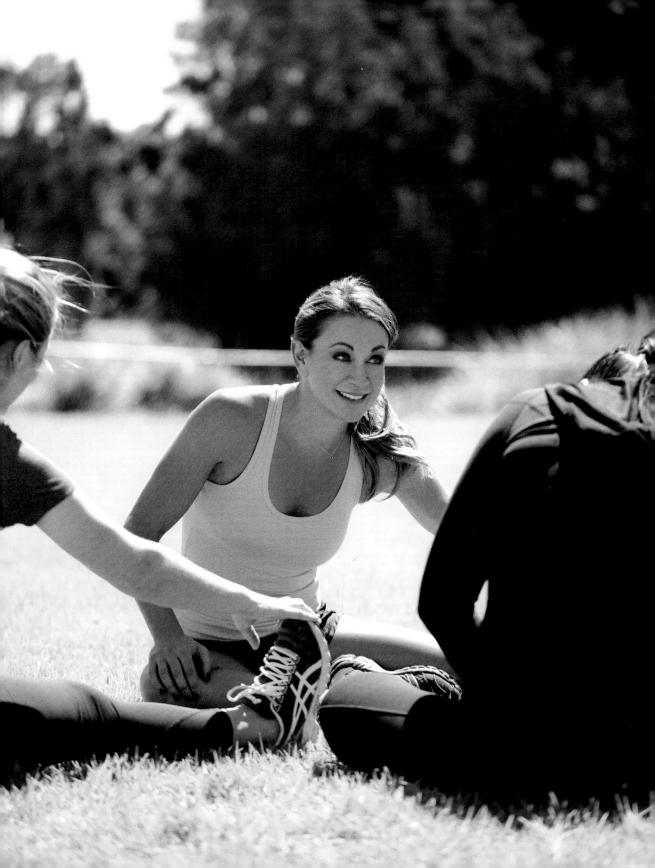

8
your exercises

"the less muscle you have, the lower your basal metabolic rate and the harder it is to burn the calories you ingest."

Okay. Here are the exercises that will change your life. You can do almost all of them at home, with minimal equipment. (For those who do use gym equipment, I note non-gym alternatives.) In the next chapter I combine them in your twelve-week workout program. First, though, I need to explain why weight training is as crucial to weight loss as your cardio workouts.

weight training rocks

Much of the weight lost with fad diets is water and muscle. Because muscle is your body's very own fat-burning furnace, your weight loss opportunities will be severely compromised without it. The less muscle you have, the lower your basal metabolic rate and the harder it is to burn the calories you ingest. Got it?

You'll need to use all the resources you can because your body will, in fact, conspire *against* you losing weight! This is because our bodies don't have a built-in level of fat that they try to maintain. Fat levels are entirely guided by how much fat we habitually store in our bodies through our diet and lifestyle. When we've been storing fat for a few years at a certain level, our bodies naturally develop all the nerves, hormones, capillaries, and connective tissue to support it. When you start to change all this by losing weight, your body quickly slips into defensive mode because it thinks that it's under threat of starvation. Your metabolism will slow down, your appetite will increase, and *your body will start trying to store more fat*. This is especially the case when you lose weight quickly, because even though you think you *gained* the weight quickly, you actually didn't. No, no, no. That backside of yours has been in the making for some time. Weight gain tends to take place over a period of years, so it's hard to sneak past your body's survival mechanisms when stripping off fat quickly.

I see a lot of people desperate to lose weight *wasting their time* with exercises that aren't suited to a weight loss program. To understand why, you need to appreciate the difference between compound and isolation exercises.

Compound exercises use more than one muscle group. Think about it—when you climb a set of stairs you:

1. Raise your right leg, flex your ankle, and plant it on the step (hello, hip flexor, quads, tibialis)

2. Push yourself up to the next step (say g'day to quadriceps, hamstrings, gluteals, calf muscles, abdominals, lower back muscles)

3. Repeat for the left leg

That simple motion has recruited over 50 percent of your body's musculature. Now compare that to one of those seated abductor/adductor machines, which uses just *two* muscles! Which one do you think will fast-track you to "hot momma"?

Isolation exercises, on the other hand, do just that—they isolate a particular muscle so that you can work *only* that muscle. This is fine if you're a bodybuilder, are training for a sports-specific purpose, or are undertaking rehabilitation training for a broken limb or whatever. But when you want to lose weight, you need to burn as many calories as you can in your workout, and the way to do that is to get as many muscles involved as possible.

All of the exercises that I give you will be compound exercises because they simply burn more calories. So if you're looking around the gym and see a personal trainer hovering over a weight loss candidate doing some crazy one-legged circus act, look on in sympathy. Then get into your compound exercises.

keep it simple

I'm frequently asked what exercises I do in my workouts, and I'm here to tell you that I keep it very, very simple. For example, there are just four elements to my leg workouts: squats, lunges, step-ups, and various forms of cardio training. For my upper body I use mainly chin-ups, push-ups, bench presses, and shoulder presses. I incorporate variations to improve muscle tone and to avoid getting stale in my workouts, but that's pretty much it.

From the thousands of exercises available, I have selected the ones that I have found to be the *most effective for weight loss and overall athletic fitness*. Basic exercises are usually the best because they have a proven track record and are easier to do. I have also selected exercises that can be done either in the gym, where there's a full range of equipment, or at home, with minimal equipment. I have provided an easier version and a harder version for some. The harder version usually uses more than just body weight. And you *must* start upping the weight if you want to lose the weight. So *keep challenging yourself*!

you gotta train hard

The next thing we need to be clear about is intensity. When you train, you must *train hard*. Watchers of *The Biggest Loser* will know just how hard those guys go, so use their efforts as a benchmark for your own. Intensity is the one thing just about everyone gets wrong. Half of the fitness industry is so busy dreaming up different programs and variations of exercises that they've forgotten that what really changes bodies is grunting and sweating!

Your heart rate will tell you how hard you're going. The first two weeks of training is simply about routine, about getting into the habit of building your fitness. In saying that, still shoot for around 65–70 percent of your maximum heart rate (MHR). See page 62 for how to calculate your MHR.

The next step is to start ramping up your workouts with bursts of 85 percent MHR. Once you're in the 70–80 percent range, your cardiovascular system is really starting to kick in.

personal trainers

I totally recommend getting a personal trainer. Make sure you get someone who is going to kick your ass. And no excuses or whining from you. Have that person coach you through the exercises I give you in this section of the book. Get your trainer to show you how to do them safely and with intensity so that you know you are not wasting your time. Suck your trainer dry about technique, why the exercises are done that way, and about safety. A good trainer should set you up so that ultimately you can go it alone.

I do, though, have a problem with personal trainers who pull out the old "muscle weighs more than fat" when you get on the scale after three weeks of training and haven't lost any weight (or, worse yet, have put it on). Muscle does, in fact, weigh more than fat; however, an overweight, unconditioned person will never put on muscle quicker than he or she will lose fat. So if this has happened, then both of you need to take some responsibility and stop wasting each other's time. You need to clean up your diet and stop rewarding yourself with food, and your trainer needs to push you harder and ensure that you're training hard when you're on your own. You must meet each other halfway.

Of course, I have omitted a lot of exercises. This book is for those who want to lose weight, burn calories, and change their body shape, and that's exactly what these basic compound exercises do. It's not for bodybuilders.

warm up and stretch down

If you are going it alone—no gym, no personal trainer—then more power to you. Remember, though, that every workout deserves a good warm-up, which can be as simple as 5 minutes on a cardio machine or a light jog around a track or the backyard. The warm-ups in your twelve-week program are based around gym equipment. But you can replace these with any jogging or jump-rope exercise that gets your heart rate to 150 by the end.

Stretches should always be done at the end of a workout, which is when they work best (unless your health practitioner recommends you do some muscle- or joint-specific stretching before your workout).

equipment checklist

- Good pair of training shoes, well-cushioned and with lateral support. It takes a week or two to break in new shoes, so have some Band-Aids around just in case. Make sure you do up your laces properly so your foot is not sliding around inside.
- For girls, a good sports bra
- Workout towel
- Water bottle
- Heart rate monitor
- Dumbbells (light to medium)
- Barbell (if you can)
- Exercise ball
- Jump rope
- Reliable alarm clock

the golden rules

The following rules apply to *every* exercise in this section. Don't forget to heed them, or you'll risk injury.

- Breathe throughout the movement—exhale on the power or pushing phase (the "concentric" phase, where the muscle is contracting), and inhale on the return phase (the "eccentric" phase, where the muscle is lengthening).
- Ensure that your knees and feet track in the same direction to avoid joint damage during knee bends.
- Soften knees and elbows by keeping them very slightly bent—never lock them straight.
- Draw in your abdominals and narrow your waist to support your back.
- Lengthen your spine by rolling your shoulders back and down and opening your chest.
- Lengthen your neck and avoid tensing it during exercise.
- Pull your chin in slightly, never letting your head roll backward.

toning exercises

I can't tell you how often I'm asked what exercises I do when I train. So, welcome to my office.

Weight training defines and reshapes your body, so I refer to it as toning. In each week of the twelve-week exercise program detailed in Chapter 9, I include two days of toning workouts, which use a combination of the exercises below. There are *stacks* of strength training exercises to choose from, so I've selected some of my favorites. Most require weights (dumbbells or barbells), but a few simply use body weight as the resistance. It would be best to join a gym for your weight training, but if you have the space at home and are very organized and motivated, you *could* get by with an exercise mat, an exercise ball, a barbell, and some dumbbells.

toning: lower body

For all the exercises in this section, remember the golden rules: chest elevated, shoulders rolled back and down, abs pulled in, neck long, and chin in slightly. Once you become familiar with the exercises, you can spice up your workout by challenging yourself with a little *variation*. Rhythm changes and bottom halves are great variations for squats, lunges, and push-ups.

Rhythm changes are just what they sound like. In squats, for example, instead of just squatting down and up at the same pace, try varying the rhythm by going down slowly to, say, the count of three, and then up quicker to a count of one. This is called a three/one.

The variations are infinite—you can do a four/one, a two/two, a four/four, and so on. So if, for example, you were doing three sets of squats, you can make the first one a two/two, the next one a three/one, and the last one a four/four.

Bottom halves: These are where you repeat the bottom half of a movement (the hardest part) several times before completing a set. They're a great way to add a whole new layer of intensity to a set. For example, let's say you normally perform ten reps in the squat, but you've decided to test yourself by making them a bit harder (good on you!). So, you get through reps number 7, 8, 9, and finally reach number 10, but this time, rather than coming all the way up to your full standing height, you only come up halfway, and then lower yourself back down to a full squat position again. You then proceed to knock out 4 or 5 more such "half reps" before finally rising all the way back up and racking the weight. As you can imagine, it's intense, but worth every extra drop of sweat!

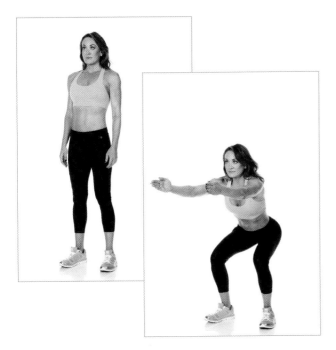

freestanding body-weight squat

1. Stand tall with your heels hip width apart, your feet slightly angled out, and your arms by your sides.
2. Imagine you are about to take a seat. Inhale as you bend your legs, and lower your hips until your thighs are almost parallel to the floor. At the same time extend your arms forward. At the bottom of the movement your knees should not be farther forward than your toes and your chest should be proud.
3. Exhale as you push through your heels, squeeze your butt, and return to the start position without locking your knees.

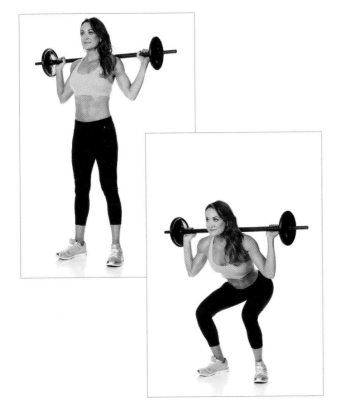

barbell squat

1. Stand tall with your heels slightly wider than hip width apart and your feet slightly angled out. Place the barbell on the fleshy part of your upper back and let the tension you feel between your shoulder blades help support the bar.
2. Inhale as you bend your legs and lower your hips until your thighs are almost parallel to the floor. Your knees should not be farther forward than your toes. Keep your chest proud and your back long.
3. Exhale as you push through your heels and squeeze your butt to return to the start position. Use a mirror, if you can, to check that your knees stay in line with your toes.

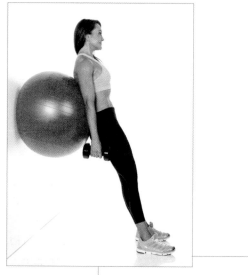

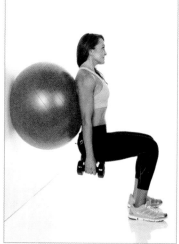

exercise ball squat

1. Place an exercise ball between you and a wall so the ball is comfortably supporting your lower back. Step your feet forward and shoulder width apart so that your heels are wider than your hips and your feet slightly angled out. Let your arms hang by your sides. If you're using dumbbells, grip them firmly.
2. Inhale as you bend your legs, and lower your hips until your thighs are almost parallel to the floor. At the bottom of the movement your knees should not be farther forward than your toes. Because you're leaning against the ball your body will remain upright.
3. Exhale as you push through your heels and squeeze your butt to return to the start position.

Variations

- Exercise ball squat with dumbbells. This will make you work even harder.
- Exercise ball squat with wide stance. This will recruit the muscles in your inner thighs more—just be sure that your knees go in the same direction as your feet, which should be pointing out slightly.

"squats are my all-time favorite leg exercise. you'll get great legs and a tight butt, and you'll burn off calories like crazy!"

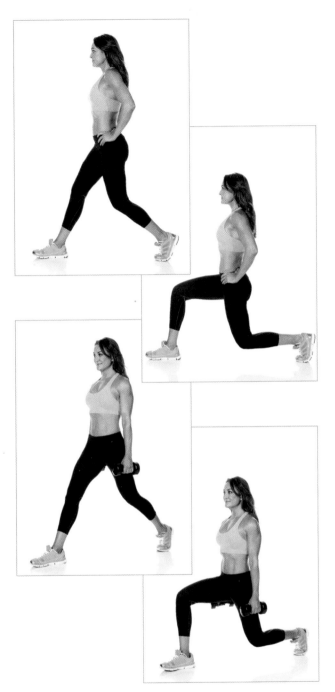

static lunge

1. Stand tall, hands on hips, and take a long step back, keeping your feet hip width apart for balance. Keep your weight evenly distributed on both legs, your front knee slightly bent, and your weight on the ball of your back foot (the heel is up). Your feet will stay in this position for the whole exercise, so make sure you feel balanced.
2. Keeping the body tall, inhale as you bend your back knee toward the floor. Try to make a right angle with each leg—the front knee should remain above the ankle and not shoot forward past it. If this happens, you need to lengthen your stride.
3. Inhale as you come up, pushing up through the front heel to engage your butt. Your movement should be up and down—*not* forward and backward.

Note: You are not "stepping" with this exercise—your feet remain static.

Variations

- A supported static lunge is good for beginners. Stand next to a bench, chair, or fence at waist height, and use one hand to steady yourself as you drop into the lunge.
- A static lunge with dumbbells or barbell really ups the ante. But don't use these until you've practiced stacks of lunges first.

"don't lean forward as you move down, and watch that front knee—make sure it doesn't drift forward past your toes."

forward power lunge

1. Stand tall, hands on hips, looking straight ahead.
2. Inhale and take a long step forward, keeping your feet hip width apart and your weight evenly distributed between your front and back legs. *Both* legs should be bent at an angle of 90 degrees.
3. Exhale and powerfully push off your front foot to get you back to start position. Repeat for the opposite leg and then alternate legs, or do several reps on one side before you swap.

Variations

- Try a forward power lunge with dumbbells.
- A backward power lunge will improve your technique.

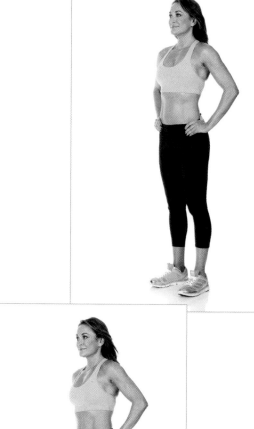

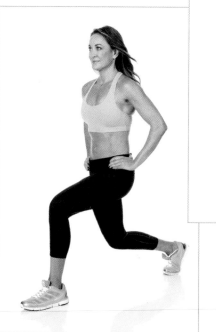

dynamic lunge

1. Find a low, solid platform around 6–12 inches high (e.g., a step) and stand on it.
2. Take a long step back, keeping your feet hip width apart and the heel of your back foot up. Both legs should be bent at 90 degrees.
3. Push off your back foot, tap the step with it, and step back again. Repeat with the same leg several times, then swap. To help with your balance, use your arms as if you are running.

Variation

- Dynamic lunge with dumbbells. The added weight will really test your balance, so slow down.

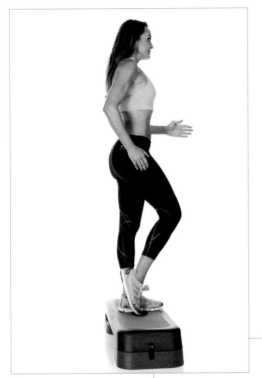

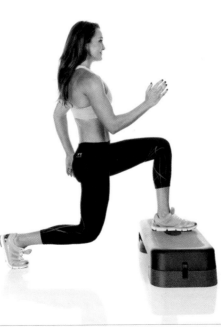

"lunges will shred your legs like there's no tomorrow!"

step-ups

1. Stand tall in front of a low bench or chair. Optional: hold medium-heavy weights in each hand. Best to try this exercise without weights until you feel you've mastered the mechanics.
2. Step your right foot up onto the bench, placing it flat.
3. Push up through the right leg and hips to place the left foot on the bench.
4. Now step back down with the right foot followed by the left. Repeat in the same order. Maintain the start position posture perfectly throughout.

Variations
- Wear a backpack with a medicine ball in it.
- Try step-ups using a high bench and weights, but don't use weights the first time—they can be a bit scary if you trip.

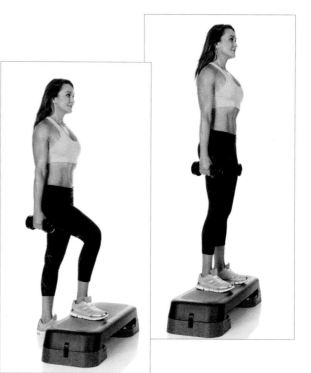

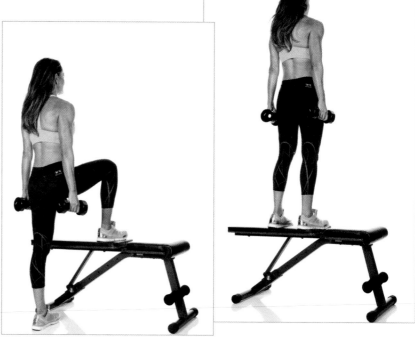

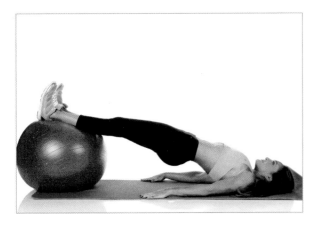

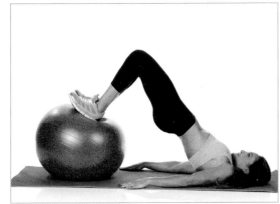

exercise ball hamstring curl

1. Lie on the floor with your arms beside you, palms facing down. Place your heels and calf muscles on the exercise ball. Have your feet about hip width apart, and flex your toes back toward you. Lift your hips up off the floor and lock your midsection tight so that your body is straight and is supported by your shoulders.

2. Keeping your torso strong, bend your knees and use your heels to roll the ball toward your butt. Keep your feet flexed and squeeze the backs of your legs and your inner thighs.

3. Roll the ball back to the start position, keeping your body taut.

"a great exercise for the backs of your legs, and your inner thighs, too!"

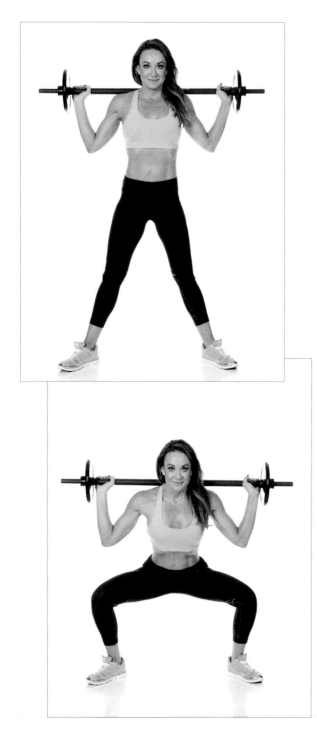

sumo squat with barbell

1. Stand with your heels widely spaced apart and your feet angled out. The wider stance means you will be using more muscles than a regular barbell squat. Place the barbell on the fleshy part of your upper back and let the tension you feel between your shoulder blades help support the bar.
2. Inhale as you bend your legs and lower your hips until your thighs are almost parallel to the floor. Keep your back strong.
3. Exhale as you push through your heels and return to the start position.

Access to a gym? You could use the leg press machine instead.

toning: upper body—back

In all of the "pulling" exercises, which we mostly perform when working the back muscles, the emphasis can be shifted simply by changing your grip on the bar. Traditionally, wide grips are most commonly prescribed by trainers, but you can also use a medium or narrow grip, or you can change your hand position from a palms-forward (overhand) to a palms-facing (underhand) grip. Is one hand position more effective than another? Not really—they all work the back muscles.

Put simply, overhand and underhand grips partially flex the lats from the start position. The best thing to do is to try them—do a set of each and you will feel the shift in emphasis and you'll also feel different muscles chipping in to help out (for example, an underhand grip will also recruit your biceps). Most important, all of these variations are "compound," which means you're working lots of muscles at the same time—*exactly* what you want for maximum calorie burning.

bent-over fly

1. Stand with your feet shoulder width apart. Bend at the waist so that your torso is approximately 45 degrees to the floor. Hold the dumbbells straight down with your arms slightly bent.
2. Exhale as you raise your arms to the side until your hands are level with your shoulders. Keep your back strong.
3. Inhale and lower your arms back to the starting position.

Access to a gym? Do lat pull-downs with a wide grip (always bring the bar to the front of your body, never behind).

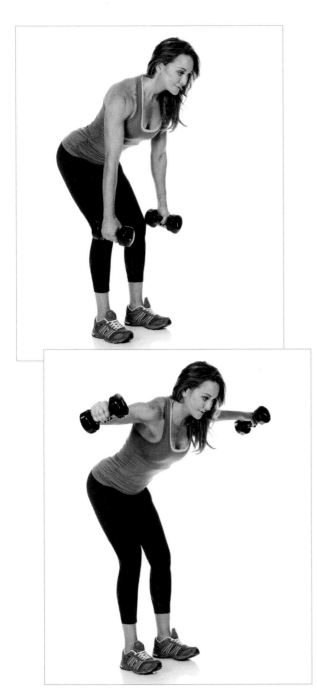

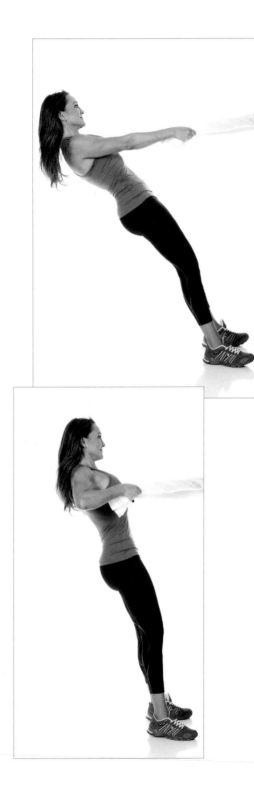

towel pulls

1. Take a towel and loop it around a fixed pole or tree at chest height. Alternatively, get a friend to hold it. Grasp one end of the towel in each hand and place your feet near the base of the pole, shoulder width apart. Lean back, letting the towel take your body weight.
2. Brace your abs, lift your chest, and exhale as you pull yourself toward the pole, tucking your elbows in and squeezing your shoulder blades together.
3. Pause, inhale, and control your return to the start position.

Variation
- Make it harder by putting on a heavy backpack.

Access to a gym? Do assisted chins. For beginners, start with a weight that represents approximately 70 percent of your body weight.

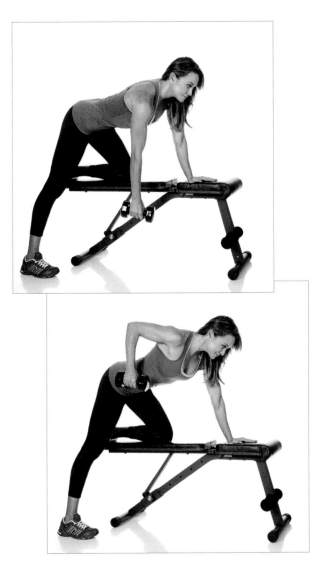

dumbbell rows

1. Select a medium-heavy dumbbell and place one knee on a bench or chair. Support yourself by placing your free hand on the bench or chair and your other foot on the ground. Square up your shoulders and hips and lock yourself into a strong position with a long, straight back. Allow the dumbbell to hang directly below your shoulder.
2. Exhale as you pull the dumbbell up to your hip, keeping your elbow close to your torso and parallel to the floor.
3. Pause, then inhale as you lower the dumbbell back to the start position. (In the workouts section later, I'll always expect you to do 15 repetitions with your left arm, followed by 15 with your right.)

"think of this one as practice for starting your lawnmower—hold your core strong and avoid twisting through the shoulders and hips."

These six exercises are great for building upper body strength and are easy to do either at home or in the gym.

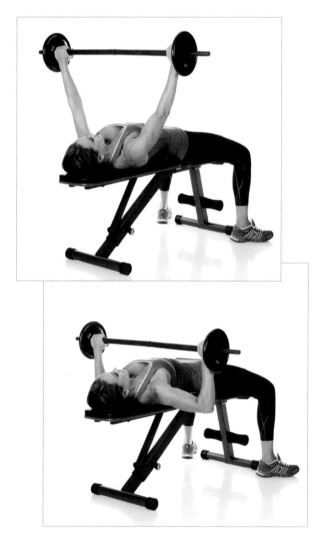

chest press with barbell

1. Lie on the floor (or on a bench) and, with arms outstretched and your hands slightly wider than shoulder width apart, grip the barbell above your chest in line with your nipples. Your feet can be either on the bench or on the ground. (You may be more stable on the ground, but you'll need to be careful not to arch your back. Do whatever works best for you.)
2. Keep your midsection braced and inhale as you lower the barbell to about 4 inches above your chest.
3. Keep your chest elevated and exhale as you press the barbell back to the start position.

Variation

• A chest press with barbell on an incline bench will work different muscles.

"this is another exercise where it's easy to hurt your shoulders, so always keep the bar over your chest, never over your face."

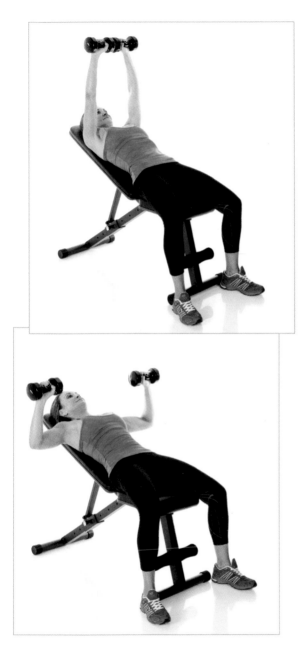

chest press with dumbbells

1. Lie on a bench or on the ground (I'm on an incline bench in the picture) and, with straight arms, hold the dumbbells firmly above your shoulders around 4 inches apart. Your feet can be either on the bench or on the ground.
2. Keep your midsection braced and inhale as you lower the dumbbells toward the outside of your chest.
3. Keep the chest proud and abs pulled in as you exhale and press the dumbbells back to the top, finishing with them about 4 inches apart.

Variations

● This exercise is great whether you're on the floor, on a flat bench, or on an incline bench at a gym.

"both arms work independently, so you may discover one side of your body is stronger than the other (very common); this exercise will help to correct it."

"exercise ball work is really challenging because of the instability—every muscle has to fire up to keep your balance!"

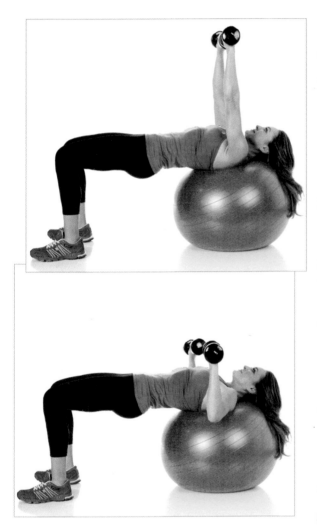

chest press with dumbbells on exercise ball

1. Sit on the edge of the exercise ball and rest some light-medium dumbbells on your thighs. Walking your feet forward, roll down the exercise ball and lower your shoulders so that your body is horizontal.
2. Lift the dumbbells above your head, holding them approximately 4 inches apart with straight arms.
3. Keep your midsection braced and inhale as you lower the dumbbells toward the outside of your chest.
4. Exhale as you press the dumbbells back to the top, keeping them 4 inches apart.

"make sure that the exercise ball is 'anti-burst' and not damaged."

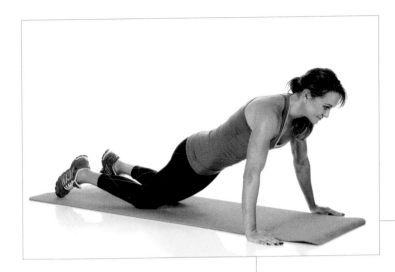

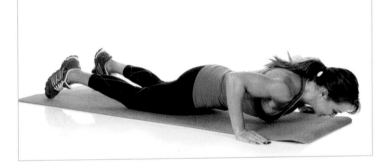

"there's a good reason why not many people can do full-length push-ups—you have to be strong!"

push-ups on knees

1. Kneel on the ground and walk your hands forward until they are slightly wider than shoulder width apart. Straighten your arms, keep your torso long and strong, and look directly ahead at the floor. Your knees can be hip width apart or together.

2. Keeping your abs pulled in, inhale, bend your elbows, and lower your upper body until your chest is about 4 inches off the floor.

3. Exhale as you straighten your arms to return to the start position.

"drop your shoulders down away from your ears, and keep your butt down—at the bottom of the movement your hands and elbows should be aligned with your chest."

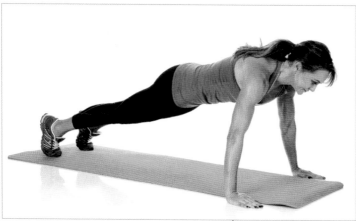

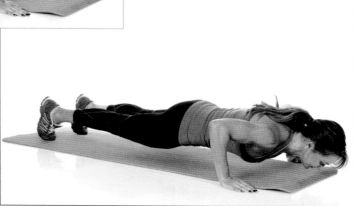

push-ups on toes

1. With your arms straight and slightly wider than shoulder width apart, support your body on hands and toes. Your toes can be hip width apart or together.
2. Inhale as you bend your arms and lower your upper body (keeping it strong and straight) until your chest is about 4 inches off the floor.
3. Exhale as you straighten your arms to return to the start position.

Variations

- Place your hands on a bench and your knees or feet on the floor.
- Place your feet on a bench and your hands on the floor.

walking push-ups with one hand elevated

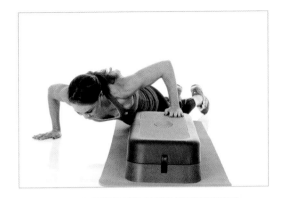

1. This exercise can be performed either on your knees or on your toes (advanced).
2. Place one hand on the end of a low bench and the other hand on the floor. Your hands should be slightly wider than shoulder width apart. Lengthen your torso, draw your abs in, expand your chest, and drop your shoulders down away from your ears. Keep your neck long and your chin tucked in, and look at the floor directly ahead.
3. Bend your arms and inhale as you lower your upper body to about 4 inches off the floor.
4. Exhale as you straighten your arms to return to the start position, then hold your body strong as you swap hands to the other side and alternate the push-up.

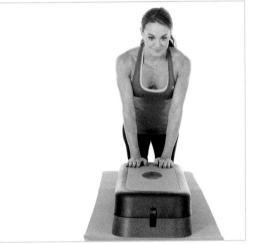

Variations

- Walking push-ups on floor (i.e., without using a low bench)
- Walking push-ups with medicine ball. Place one hand on a medicine ball, perform 1 rep, then roll it across to your other hand and perform another one, and so on. Great stuff!

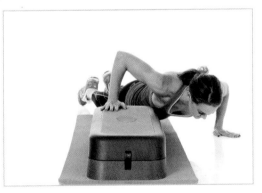

"the 'walking' component really smashes core muscles; you can 'walk' your body after each repetition or perform 3 to 5 reps on each side before swapping."

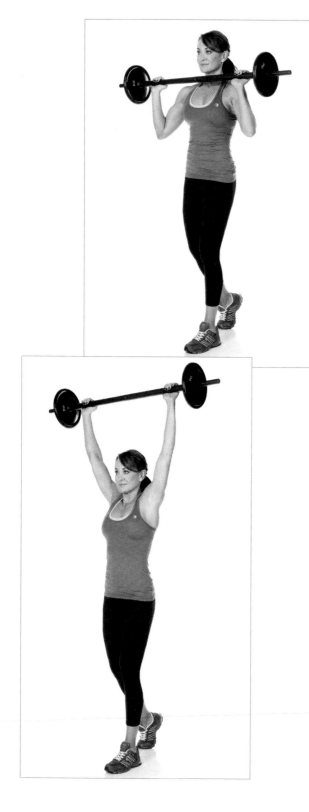

Let's face it—everyone loves a good set of shoulders! The exercises in this section are my faves for upper body strength in the arms and shoulders.

standing shoulder press

1. Holding a barbell (or dumbbells), stand tall with your feet in a staggered stance. Your front knee should be soft and take most of your body weight; the ball of your back foot should be on the floor, your back leg acting as a prop to stop you from leaning backward. You should feel rock solid.
2. Keeping your midsection braced, exhale as you drive the barbell toward the ceiling, keeping it slightly forward of your face at the top of the movement. Do not lock your elbows, keep them slightly bent. And *do not* push the bar back behind your head (or I will beat you and then give you my chiropractor's number).
3. Inhale as you carefully lower the barbell to the start position. Look forward throughout the movement and take care not to arch your back.

Variation

- Standing shoulder press with dumbbells. Hold the dumbbells close to the shoulders, then exhale as you drive them toward the ceiling, aiming them to finish about 4 inches apart.

standing biceps curl with barbell

1. Holding the barbell in a natural carrying position, stand tall with one foot forward and one back. Your front knee should be soft and the ball of your back foot acting as a prop to stop you from leaning backward.
2. Exhale as you raise the bar to your upper chest, keeping your upper arms parallel with your body and your elbows in. Avoid letting the bar collapse against your chest.
3. Keeping the midsection tight, inhale as you lower the bar to the start position. Your upper arms should remain still. Do not let your elbows point behind you on the way down or in front of you on the way up. The only direction they should be pointing is *down*. Keep your body still and avoid rocking or swaying.

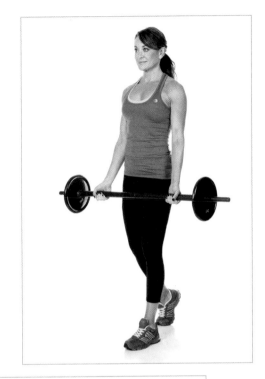

"the most common mistake here is slouching and letting your shoulders roll over. keep your chest up!"

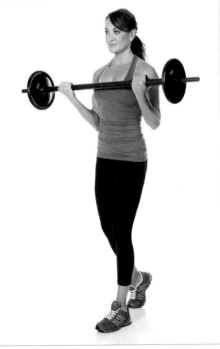

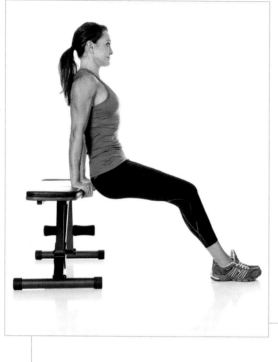

triceps bench dips

1. Sit on a low bench and grip the edge. Support your weight through your arms and shoulders and walk your legs forward so that your thighs are parallel to the floor and your feet are flat.
2. Inhale as you lower your body until your upper arms are almost horizontal.
3. Exhale as you drive yourself up to the start position, contracting the muscles in the back of your arms.

Variations
- Put your feet on another bench.
- Increase the resistance further by placing a medicine ball or weight plate on your lap.

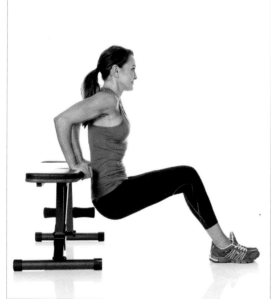

"you should feel punished after dips. I've had my heart rate at 163 with this exercise!"

The main focus with all abdominal training is to pull or draw your abs inward throughout the entire movement, both up and down. Think of "narrowing" the waist rather than "thickening" it.

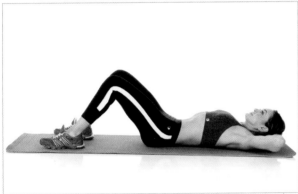

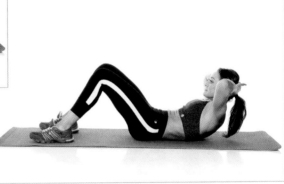

crunch

1. Lie on the floor and bend your knees so that your feet are flat on the floor. Draw in your abs, narrowing your waist, and place your hands palms down beside you, across your chest, or—the hardest option—behind your head. (If your hands are behind your head, keep your elbows out of sight and avoid pulling on your head and bending your neck.)
2. Keeping your abs tight, exhale as you roll or "crunch" your upper torso. Keep your chin in and look forward.
3. Keep your abs drawn in and inhale as you lower yourself back down to the start position.

Variation
- Crunch with medicine ball. Holding a medicine ball increases the intensity.

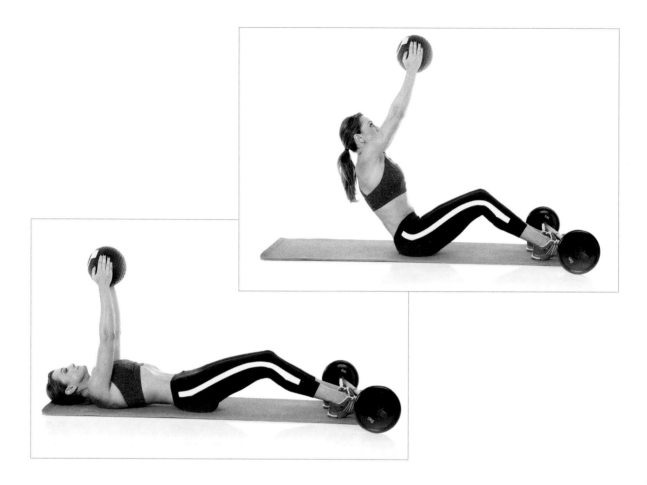

supported crunch with medicine ball

1. Sit on the floor and tuck your feet under a support such as a weighted bar, a ledge, or even the edge of your couch. Bend your knees to 90 degrees and roll back, lying flat and holding the medicine ball directly above your chest.
2. Exhale as you lift your body upward toward the ceiling.
3. Drawing the abs in tight, inhale and lower yourself down to the start position.

Variations

- Supported crunch without medicine ball. Using the medicine ball really challenges, so start off without it if it's too much.
- Supported crunch with twist. Lift one shoulder to the opposite knee for several repetitions, or alternate.

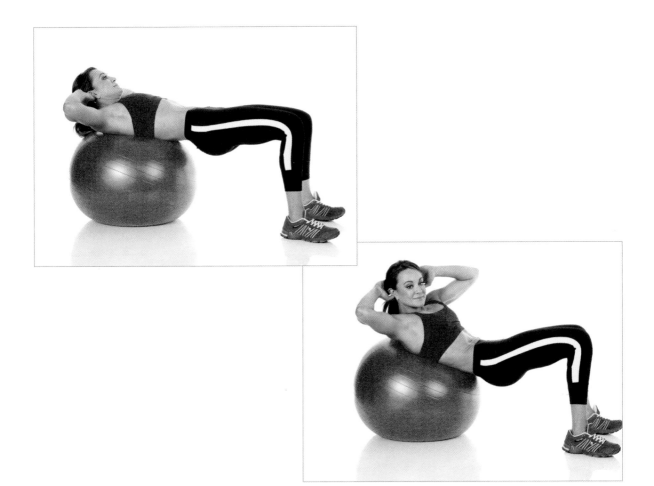

exercise ball crunch with twist

1. Sit on the exercise ball and roll yourself down until it's under your lower back, and your thighs and torso are parallel with the floor. Draw your abs inward, narrowing your waist, and place your hands either across your chest or behind your head.
2. Exhale as you raise your body up to an angle of around 45 degrees, adding a twist by lifting one shoulder toward the opposite leg.
3. Keeping your abs pulled in, inhale and lower yourself back down to the start position.

Variations
- Exercise ball crunch with medicine ball. Try it without the twist first.
- Lift the opposite leg off the floor during the twist to really test your balance.

"try to aim your knees at the roof rather than bringing them to your chest—keep your chin in and your head on the floor."

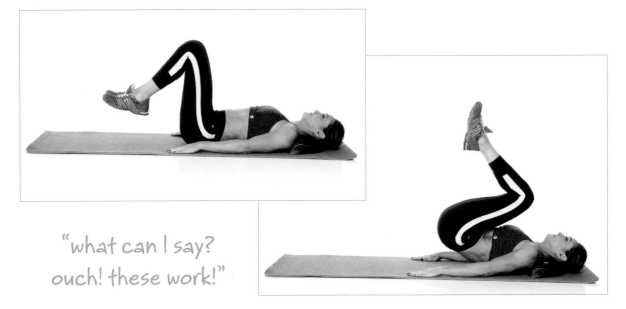

"what can I say? ouch! these work!"

reverse crunch

1. Lie on your back and bend your knees, inhaling as you lift your legs so that your thighs are at 90 degrees and directly over your hips. Draw your abdominals down to hollow out the belly and keep your lower back firm against the floor. Place your arms beside you, palms down.
2. Exhale as you lift the lower half of your body toward the ceiling.
3. Inhale as you lower carefully to your start position.

Note: Stay away from "swinging" the legs. Rather, it's a small and intense squeeze and lift.

double crunch

1. Lie on your back and lift your legs above you, keeping your knees bent at 90 degrees and directly over your hips. Hollow out your belly so that your lower back is firm against the floor, and place your hands behind your head.
2. Exhale as you lift the upper and lower halves of your body at the same time. Think of squeezing yourself into a tiny ball. Keep your elbows out and avoid pulling on your head.
3. Inhale as you uncurl back to the start position, going slowly to protect your back.

Note: there's no photo for this, but just add the crunch (page 99) and reverse crunch (this page) together and you've got it!

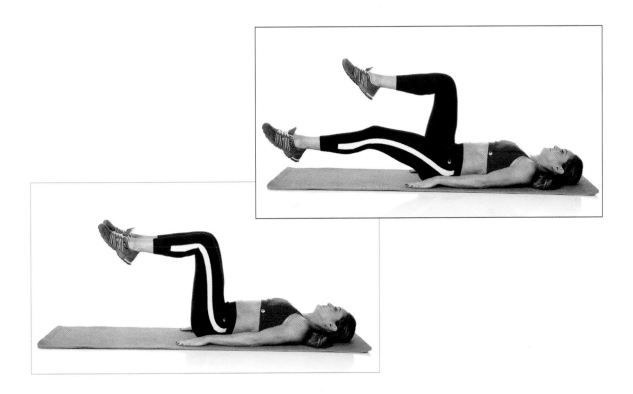

leg extensions

1. Lie on your back and lift your legs above you, keeping your knees bent at 90 degrees and directly over your hips. Place your arms beside you, palms down, and keep your lower back firm against the floor.

2. Keeping one leg in place, exhale and straighten the other leg away from you until you can no longer keep your abs drawn in. As soon as you feel your abs pop outward or your lower back start to arch away from the floor, you have extended the leg too far. Pull your leg back until you can reset your abs inward. The stronger you get, the further you will be able to extend your leg. Keep your head on the floor.

"you gotta train those abs of yours to stay in and not bulge or pop out."

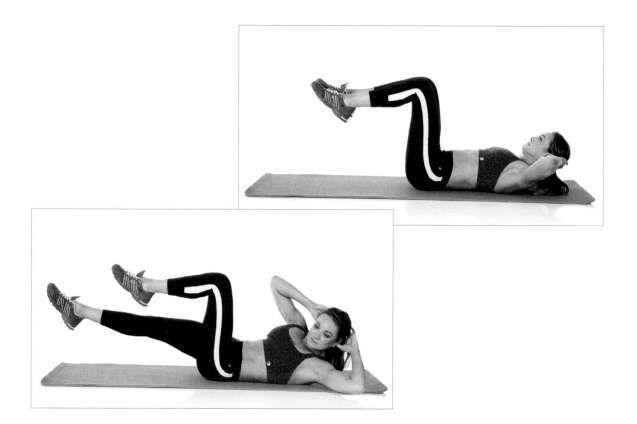

leg extensions with twisting crunch

1. Lie on your back and lift your legs above you, keeping your knees bent at 90 degrees and directly over your hips. Place your hands behind your head for support (avoid pulling and bending your neck) and keep your elbows wide and out of sight.

2. Exhale and extend one leg as you simultaneously lift the shoulder on the same side toward the bent knee. You must keep your abs pulled in throughout the entire movement. As soon as you feel your abs pop out, you have extended the leg too far, so pull your leg back to reset your abs.

lower body twist

1. Lie on your back and lift your knees over your hips. Place your arms outstretched beside you, palms down.
2. "Glue" your legs and feet together. Inhale as you slowly lower both legs to one side, to about halfway down, keeping your shoulders on the floor.
3. Exhale as you slowly drag the legs back to center.
4. Repeat on the other side.

Variation

- Increase the resistance by lowering the legs farther, or by extending the legs at an angle greater than 90 degrees.

"try to keep the upper half of your body relaxed and in perfect posture, and really wring out that waistline!"

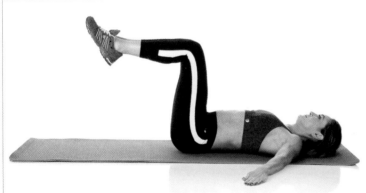

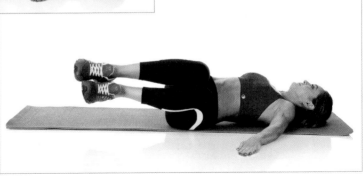

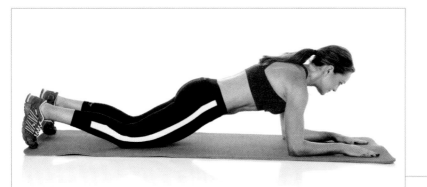

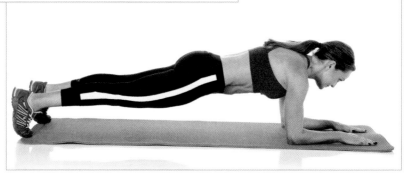

plank on knees or toes

1. Lay facedown on the floor. Place your hands forward and flat, elbows directly under your shoulders. Lengthen your neck, pull your chin in, and look at your hands. Keep your knees on the floor and hip width apart. Your body should be like a plank of wood, so keep your abs pulled in.

2. Get the feeling of pushing yourself away from the floor to stabilize your shoulders. Keep breathing steadily and easily, and keep your body in alignment. Tuck your tailbone under very slightly.

3. When you're ready to try your toes, start on your toes and stay for as long as you can before finishing the time on your knees. Work up to 1 minute.

"try not to roll forward or backward through the shoulders or hips; instead stay nice and square. you will feel the underside of your body really firing up."

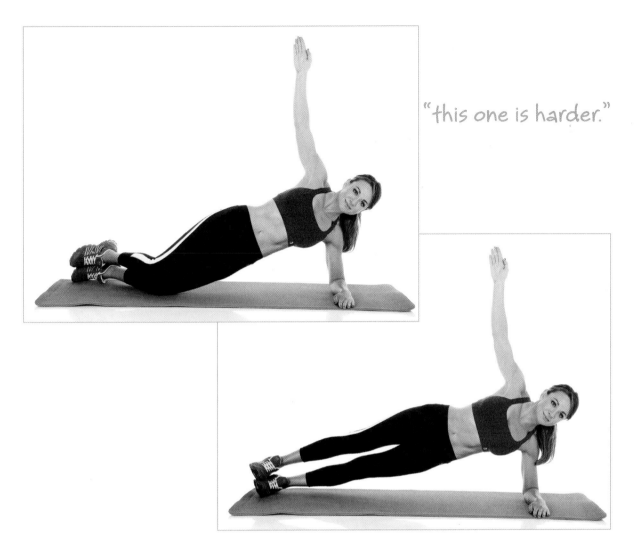

"this one is harder."

side plank

1. Lie on your side, raise yourself up on one elbow, palm flat, and "stack" your shoulders, hips, knees, and feet perpendicular to the floor. Inhale as you open up your chest, stabilizing yourself on your elbow and hip. Work from your knees to start with, bending them at 90 degrees.

2. Exhale as you lift your hip so your body is in a straight line from your knees to your head. Imagine you are pushing up out of your shoulder, which will enable you to draw the shoulders back and down and lengthen your neck.

3. Extend your other arm straight up to the roof to help you open up your chest. If you're working from your feet, keep your legs long and strong. Breathe and hold for 30 seconds to 1 minute.

I find most of my deconditioned clients really need this type of exercise, and it's often due to so many of us spending a lot of time behind a desk, or behind a wheel, which is when we tend to be lax through the upper and lower back and through the core. These exercises can be done anywhere, and you don't really need any equipment.

kneeling core and balance

1. Start on all fours with your hands directly under your shoulders and your knees directly under your hips. Draw your waistline in, pulling your belly button up.

2. Maintaining your balance, slowly reach out with your right arm long and strong as you push through the heel to extend your left leg in the opposite direction no higher than the line of the torso. You should feel like you are stretching both ways. Try to minimize wobbling by scooping up your abs and making your belly hollow.

3. Continue to move your limbs in and out slowly, really wringing out your muscles. Do several repetitions on one side before swapping. (In some workouts I get you to hold the last rep for 1 minute.)

Variation

- You can change the training effect by extending the opposite limbs out on a diagonal. This really fires up those core muscles!

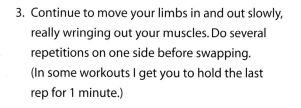

"most people are really wobbly to start with, but once you get tuned into your body, you will start to become strong and still."

"keep your toes flexed to avoid cramping in your calf."

"go slowly and really feel the squeeze through the back, butt, and back of the leg."

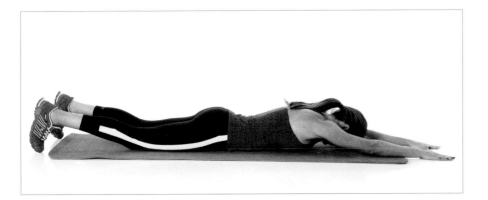

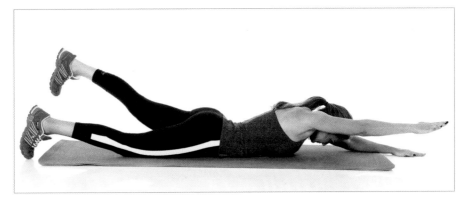

"a lot of people seem to stick their chin out and then wonder why their neck is getting sore. tuck your chin in and lengthen your neck."

alternating back extension

1. Lie on your stomach with your arms straight out in front and your legs extended behind you.
2. Exhale and slowly lift your right arm, your left leg, and your chest off the floor simultaneously. You *must* keep looking straight down at the floor with your chin pulled in and your neck relaxed (otherwise you'll hurt your neck).
3. Inhale and lower, then repeat on the opposite side.

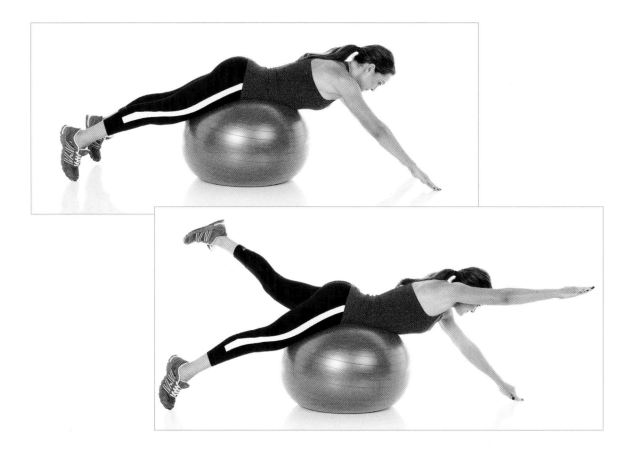

exercise ball alternating back extension

1. Drape yourself over an exercise ball on your stomach with both arms and legs extended so your toes just touch the floor to keep you balanced.
2. Exhale and slowly lift your right arm and your left leg. Remember, keep looking straight down with your chin tucked in and your neck soft.
3. Inhale and lower, then swap sides.

Variation

● Do several reps on one side before you swap.

"tuck that chin in and lengthen your neck, or you'll regret it when you wake up the next morning and you can't turn your head to turn the alarm clock off!"

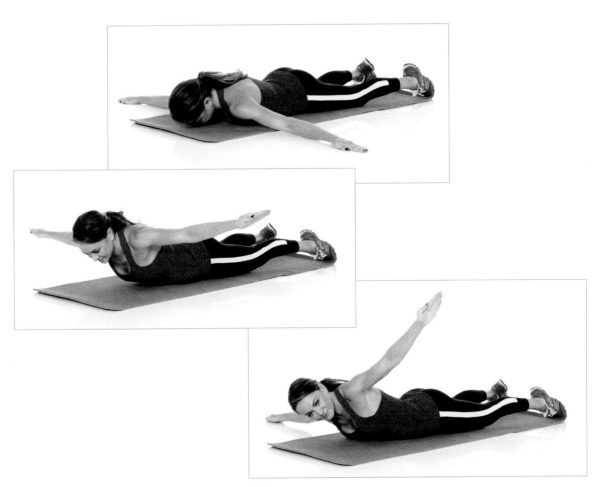

airplanes

1. Lie on your stomach with both arms outstretched at right angles, forehead on the floor and legs shoulder width apart.
2. Keeping your toes on the floor, exhale and slowly lift your upper body off the floor. You *must* keep looking straight down with your chin pulled in to avoid hurting your neck.
3. Tilt your body to one side as if you're a plane tipping its wing (keeping your neck aligned with your spine), reset to center, inhale, and lower your chest to the floor. Repeat for the opposite side.

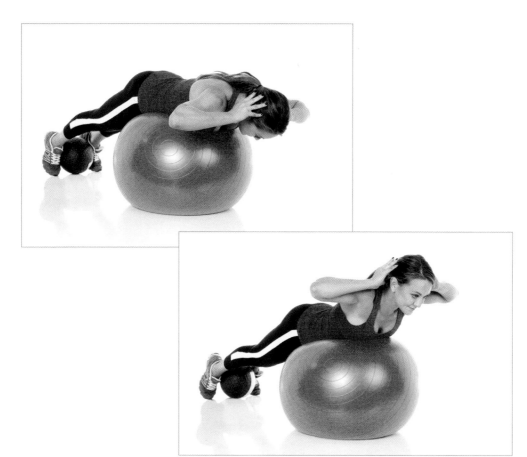

supported back extension on exercise ball

1. Drape yourself over an exercise ball on your stomach and firmly grip a medicine ball between your ankles on the floor behind you. Place your hands either out in front of you or behind your head.
2. Exhale and slowly lift your upper body. Remember, keep looking straight down with your chin tucked in and your neck soft.
3. Inhale and lower, then repeat.

fitness training

Cardiovascular fitness training is any kind of training that gets the heart rate up. Most trainers associate it with aerobic activity (running, cycling, etc.), but if you use my methods in the weight room (i.e., lots of super sets with not much rest in between), then you can be sure of getting a good cardiovascular response *whenever* you train. When your heart is pumping and you're huffing and puffing, you're burning fat—and that's why we're here! Plus, you're getting fitter, which is why I call cardio workout days your *fitness* days in the workouts in Chapter 9.

We've covered plenty of exercises with weights, so now we'll go through a few calorie-smashers you can do either outside or inside. There are hundreds of cardiovascular exercises and drills to choose from, but these are the ones that I like to use because I know they work!

running

As we discovered in Chapter 7, walking is a waste of time for weight loss unless you either start negotiating some serious hills or pump up the speed to around 4–5 miles per hour, which should have you puffing so hard that you can only say two or three words between breaths. Walking is really only a pre-cursor to the *real* calorie burners, jogging and running.

If you think you're too big to run, check out *The Biggest Loser* contestants! We've had people well over 300 pounds running within a few short weeks! So start injecting jogging into the mix. Come on! You *can* do it! Work up to, say, a 1-minute jog followed by a 2-minute walk and so on, until you can jog your entire course without stopping.

But this process has *got* to work like a ratchet. You can *never* go backward. From there improve your jogging time, and then increase the distance so that you are exercising for the same amount of time but jogging *all* the way. Now you are really chewing calories and getting fitter!

However, if you absolutely *cannot* jog or run due to a preexisting injury but you can walk, then I have the answer: get on the treadmill. First, walk as briskly as you can—at, say, 3 miles per hour—and then turn that sucker up to an incline of 15 percent. Now your cardiovascular system is working at pretty much the same level as a jog, but with virtually no impact.

In Chapter 9, you'll see that you can use jogging as your warm-up, or as your "final blast" at the end of a workout. If you are unable to get to the gym, or if someone is using your exercise space, get your running shoes on and *go*. Just make sure you go hard.

The difference between jogging and running is simply the speed at which you're traveling. Around 5 miles per hour is a jog, and anything over around 6 miles per hour is a run, but it's all relative. What I consider jogging is running for a lot of my clients, but when I jog with my friend Shannan, it's all I can do to keep up with him—it feels like sprinting to me!

Moving from brisk power-walking to jogging and then up to running takes time, but it's all doable. Jogging on grass offers more cushioning for your joints; jogging on sand is even lower impact on your joints, and it's also good for strengthening the ankles, but it's a little tougher. Jogging or running outside is *very* different from jogging or running on a treadmill, and I encourage my clients to do both. Treadmills are great, though, when it's pouring outside, and are safer for people who live in poorly lit areas but can only train at night.

My own running schedule depends on how I am feeling at the time and whether or not I have trained hard the day before. As I am writing this section of the book I am feeling very pleased with myself because this morning I got up and ran about 8 miles,

which is a lot for me! I only ran that far because yesterday was my day off, so I was feeling fresh and it was a cool autumn morning—great weather for running.

treadmills

One of my clients had only ever done her running training on the treadmill, so her first outdoor run was a shock. This was because when she ran on her treadmill at 0 percent gradient, it was the equivalent of running *downhill*. All she was doing was running to stop herself from falling over, not propelling herself forward. (To simulate running outdoors, always set the gradient on your treadmill at a minimum of 2 percent.)

My client was able to get fitter faster by adding some outdoor training to her schedule, and it also gave some freshness to her training.

setting your route

Set out a route that you feel is achievable. It might be one block around your house or it might be two laps on a track—it doesn't matter. First, take a drive around your neighborhood and watch your odometer to work out how many miles it is to the park and back, around the block, and so on. That way when you get out on the road, you'll know exactly how far you're running in each session—1 mile might be longer than you think!

Set up the course, wear your watch, and then go. Some days your focus will be about doing it in your best time; other days you will be happy with just getting the job done. Occasionally you will try to extend the course by adding another lap or two without caring about the time. Mix it up.

running technique

Watch your technique. Remember to keep your abs pulled in, chest lifted, shoulders back and down, neck long, chin in, face relaxed. Try to land softly without thumping your feet. The heel should strike the ground first and then naturally roll onto the ball of the foot. Use your legs like shock absorbers and try to keep your knees aligned with your toes, rather than having them roll or cave in. Think light. Swing your arms and get yourself into a steady rhythm.

Most of all, just stay calm and relaxed. Don't listen to the negative self-talk telling you to stop, or that you are dying. You don't have to beat any world record; you just have to go. My experience tells me that you *will* surprise yourself!

The following variations are great running drills that you can introduce into your training that will help you improve your running technique and fitness.

stair runs

Find a big flight of stairs (the more the better—at least twenty) and run up it, then walk down. Take one step at a time at first, then graduate to taking two steps at a time. You may need to hang on to the handrail until you get your confidence. Stair runs can also double as a fitness test: how long does it take you to get to the top? Try to beat your time, though always use the same flight of stairs.

hill runs

These can be done either outside or on a treadmill. Run up a hill (sand hills are fantastic if you live near any), walk back down it, and repeat. If you're using a treadmill, remember to rest your feet on the side boards as you increase the treadmill's gradient and speed. Then lower yourself onto the belt and run on a steep incline for 1 minute before jumping your feet out to the side boards and reducing the incline and the speed back down to a walk for 1 minute. Some treadmills can be programmed to do this—ask your gym staff to show you how.

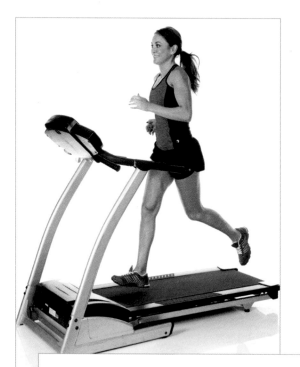

treadmill interval sprints

These can be done either outside or on a treadmill. When you're outside, sprint a specific distance, such as the length of a football field, then walk back. Time yourself, then try to beat your time.

If you're using a treadmill, rest your feet on the side boards as you increase the treadmill's speed up to your sprint speed. Supporting your weight on the side handles, lift and lower yourself onto the belt, sprint for 30 seconds, and then jump out to the sides. (Note: This is an advanced drill, so practice jumping on and off at a lower speed first!)

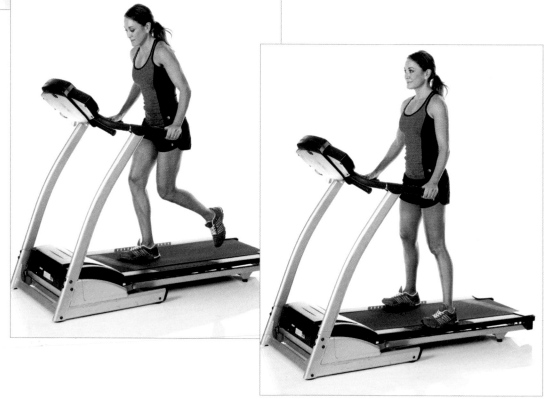

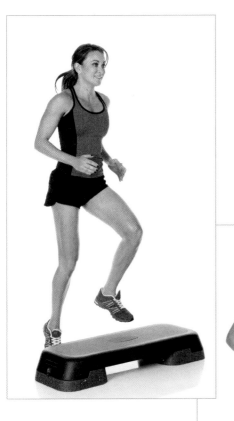

fast low-step running

Find a low step or take an aerobics step, stand in front of it, and quickly step up onto it and back down—right and left up, right and left down, right and left up, right and left down—as fast as you can for a set time or a set number of reps. Work your arms to give you more speed.

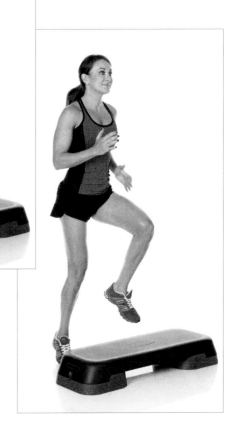

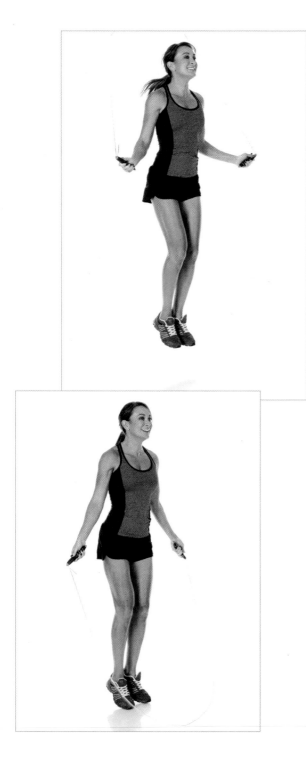

jumping rope

Jumping rope is a great way to get your heart rate up, work on your coordination, and help with your fitness. There's a good reason why boxers do it! Get yourself a jump rope and start a competition at home. Who can do the most jumps nonstop? Keep a record, stick it up on the fridge to inspire the family, and make sure someone always witnesses any attempt. You don't want any fouls called!

cycling

Cycling offers a great cardiovascular workout, but without the joint impact. For those who are very overweight or injured, cycling is a fantastic option. It is often prescribed for those who are rehabilitating from knee and hip injury or surgery.

I am a big fan of indoor classes because you can't get hit by a car and you can't fall off! Indoor bikes can do just about everything you can do outside. In fact, many professional cyclists use them for their training.

rowing machine

Rowing rocks! I advise you to get one of the gym staff to show you how to use the rower, and then just practice. I use this equipment as a great warm-up exercise and also as a fantastic cardio burst with 500-meter sprints, approximately one-third of a mile. Any time under 3 minutes for a 500-meter sprint is good. Anything under 2 minutes is *amazing*.

agility training

Being agile enables you to rapidly change direction without losing speed, balance, or control. The best thing about this type of training, which comprises lots of short, sharp movements, is that you don't need *any* equipment except a good pair of cross-trainers!

sideways running

Starting with your right foot, run three to five steps sideways to the right. On the last step your right foot should "stick" as you first drop your weight into that leg before pushing off with it and stepping out with your left. (When you plant your foot on the last step your whole foot should be in contact with the ground and slightly angled out in the direction you were heading. Make sure your knee is pointing in the same direction as your toes. Keep your shoulders back and down, with your chest up and abs in, and swing your arms to give you momentum.) The timing should feel like "one, two, drop and push, one, two, drop and push."

forward and backward jumps

With your feet hip width apart, point your toes
and knees straight ahead, keep your knees soft
like shock absorbers, pull your abs in, and elevate
your chest. Jump over a line (or a rope or towel)
and back again. Land softly!

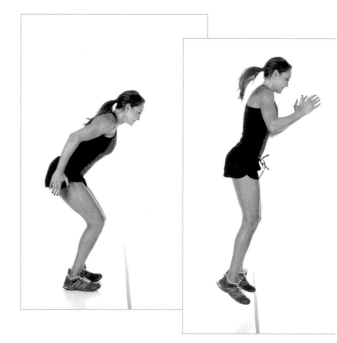

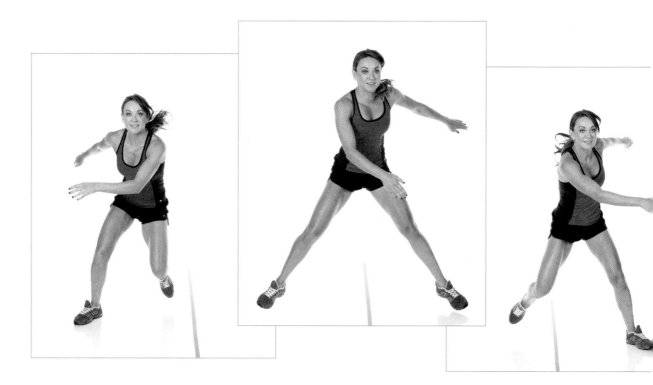

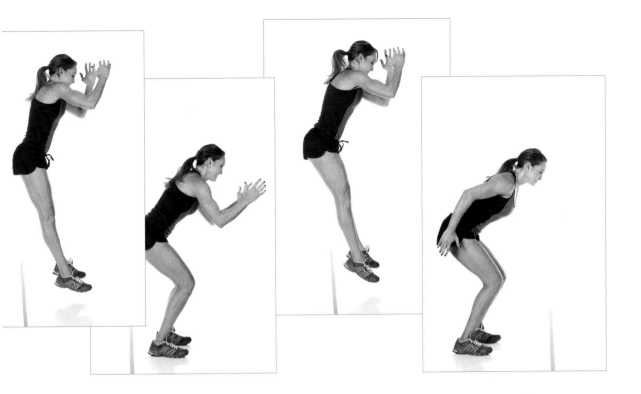

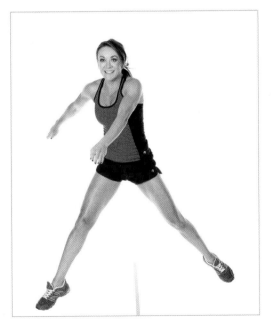

ice skaters on the spot

Lay a towel down or set up a low-step platform and take a long low leap over it sideways. Swing your arms strongly in the direction you are traveling and land the foot solidly with the toes and knee aligned (slightly angled out). Bend into the leg before you push off, leading with the other leg and repeating for the opposite side.

ski jumps

Keeping your toes and knees aligned and your knees soft, switch on your abs, lift your chest, and jump sideways over a line, towel, or rope on the ground. Pump your arms to maintain your momentum.

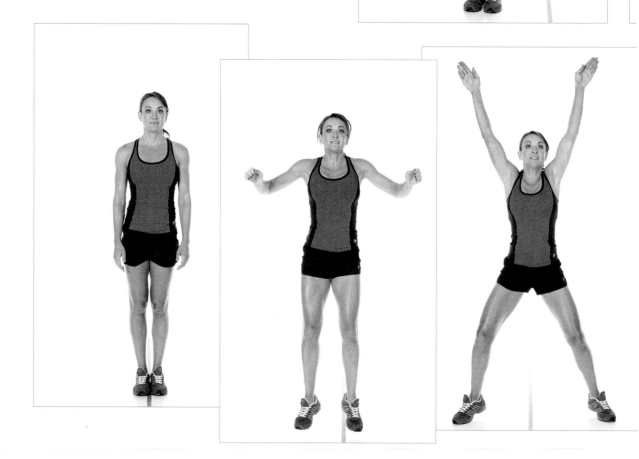

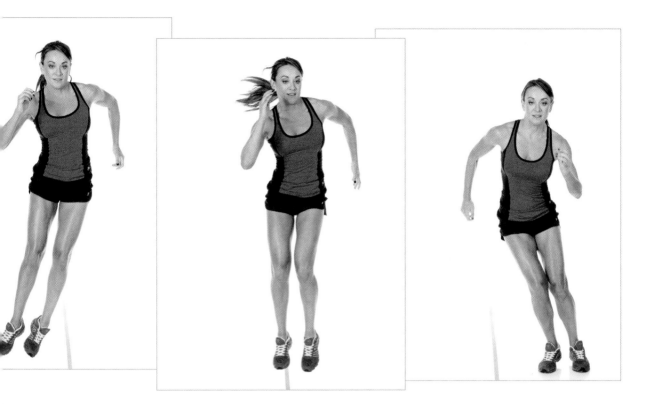

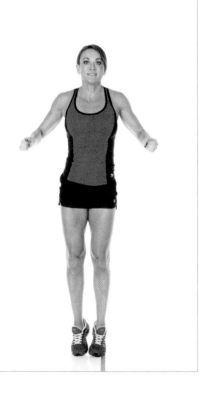

jumping jacks

Start with your feet together, then jump them about shoulder width apart. Try to land softly and have your heels contact the ground. Toes are slightly turned out, as are the knees (a lot of people seem to "cave in" their knees—ouch!), and let your legs act like shock absorbers as you jump your feet back together. Swing your arms out to the sides or overhead. Keep your abs in, chest up, and shoulders back.

basketball jumps

These are similar to jumping jacks but work from side to side. Take a low long step to the right, bend through the legs, and keep your knees aligned with your toes. Step the left foot in and spring off from both feet to shoot your basket, then repeat on the other side. Swing your arms out wide in the step, then scoop them through for the shot. The lower you go, the higher you jump.

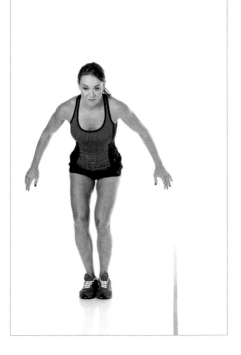

over-the-fence jumps

Take a bench and, standing on one side, bend down and grip the edges on either side. Using both feet, spring yourself up and over to the other side and then spring straight back again. Do not stop or double-bounce, and try to keep your feet together. You'll need to keep your shoulders braced to support your weight and to keep your midsection switched on.

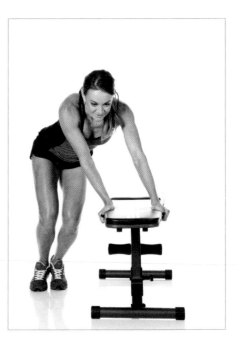

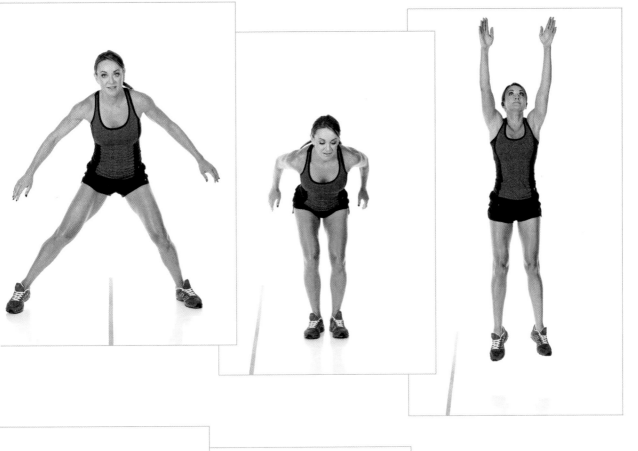

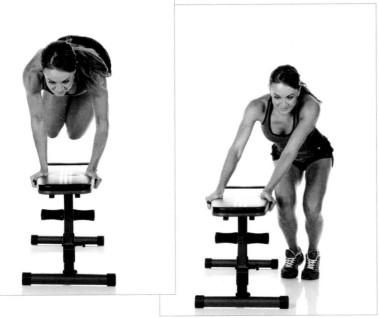

boxing

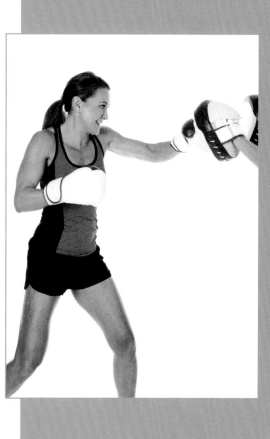

I've recently hooked up with a boxing coach and let me say this: Oh. My. God! He worked me so hard I thought I was going to bring up a lung or a kidney or both! I burned 836 calories in 50 minutes!

It's hard to do boxing on your own if you've never really done it before, and although many health clubs have equipment you can use, it's always a good idea to get some proper advice. My suggestions:

- Go to a boxing class at your health club and just join in (maybe take a friend if you are a bit nervous; that way you can partner up).
- Get a personal trainer who specializes in boxing. He or she should be able to show you how to punch the bag so that you can go at it when you're on your own.

flexibility training

In my experience, no one ever stretches enough. Stretching always seems to get thrown in at the end of a session as a token gesture—I am guilty of this myself. Stretching helps prevent injuries, and is best done after a workout when you are nice and warm. Now that I've said that, it's important to remember that this is *not* a stretching manual,

it's a weight loss manual. I also know that at this stage of the book most people will flip through a few pretty photos of stretches and say, "Yeah, whatever," and ignore the stretches themselves.

To avoid that happening, and to give you the best chance of incorporating stretching into your routine, I've put together a basic stretching sequence that loosens up all the big muscle groups. It's not a glossary of stretches—it's a sequence that starts with the large muscles and finishes with the small ones. Learn the sequence and incorporate it into the end of every training session. Once you have learned the stretches and understand the pattern you should be able to run through them in about 5 to 10 minutes.

It's definitely not the *only* way to stretch; it's just a guide to get you loosened up after your workout. And in the hustle-and-bustle world in which we live, I'll be happy if I can get you doing this much. The key here is to make sure you get to a yoga, stretch, or Body-Balance class occasionally to help loosen up your newly developed muscles—and to show off your fabulous new body!

basic stretching sequence

In the sequence below, try to hold each stretch for approximately 1 minute. Keep breathing, and try to sink deeper into the stretch as you exhale. Do not bounce into your stretches or hold your breath.

lower back stretch

Lying on the ground, roll your knees up into your chest, wrap your arms around your legs, and gently pull them in. If you can't reach around your legs, wrap a towel across your shins to pull them in.

back twist

Straighten your legs and lengthen out your body. Bring one leg up into a right angle and, using the opposite hand, gently pull your knee across your body, gently twisting your lower back. Extend the other arm out, trying to keep both shoulders on the ground. Turn your head away from the bent knee. Keep breathing, and with every exhalation gently sink deeper into the stretch. Repeat on the opposite side.

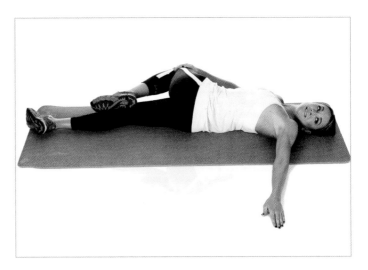

hip opener

Bring one leg up into a right angle and, leaving your foot on the floor, cross the other leg over it. Use your hand to gently press the crossed knee away to open the hip. To get more out of the stretch, reach through and clasp your hands behind your leg, then gently pull both legs toward you (pictured). If you can't reach, use a towel. If it's quite easy to reach and you want to increase the stretch, lace your hands in front of your shin. Repeat on the opposite side.

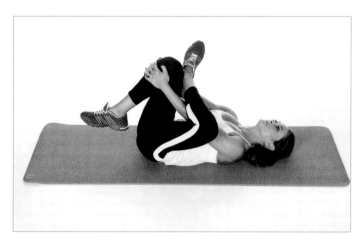

hamstring stretch

Keeping one leg bent with the foot flat on the ground, bring the other leg toward you. Clasp your hands behind your knee (or calf if you can) and lift your leg and point it to the ceiling. Keep it slightly bent and flex your foot, and you will feel the stretch in your hamstring. Again, if you need to, wrap a towel around your calf or shoe to gently pull your leg toward you. Increase the stretch effect by straightening the base leg out. Repeat on the opposite side.

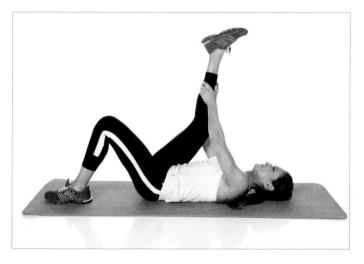

child's pose

With your knees shoulder width apart, slide your buttocks back onto your heels and extend your arms in front, lowering your forehead toward the ground. In yoga this is known as "child's pose."

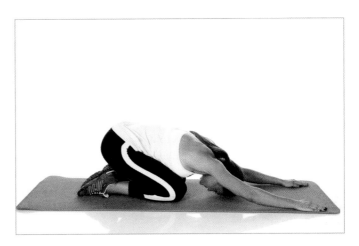

inner thigh stretch

1. These are particularly good if you are doing a lot of running. Kneel on all fours and, keeping your arms straight, extend your leg out to the side with your foot pointing forward.
2. Uncurl the toes on your supporting leg and slowly sit your butt down, dropping onto your elbows at the same time. Feel the stretch running down the inside of your straight-leg thigh.
3. Return to all fours, straightening your arms and stepping the leg back before repeating on the other side.

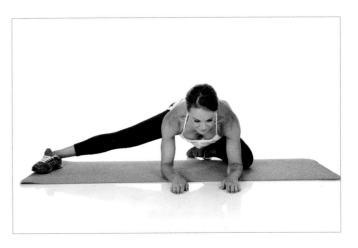

quadriceps stretch

Stand tall and, extending one arm for balance, curl your leg up behind you and grab your foot with the same hand. Keeping your knees together, gently pull your heel into your butt. Draw your abs in and pull your shoulders back and down, elevating your chest. Think about tucking your tailbone under to get more of a stretch. If your balance is good, put both hands behind you and hold your foot, fully expand your chest, and pull your shoulders back. Repeat on the opposite leg.

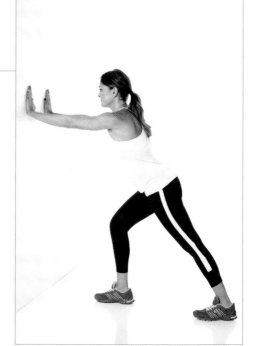

calf stretch

Push against a solid wall or railing and step one foot back. Keep the toes of the back foot pointing straight ahead and push the heel into the ground. Now lean into the wall to feel the stretch in the upper calf. Bend the back knee to deepen the stretch.

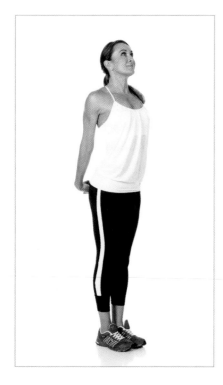

chest stretch

Stand tall, draw your abs in, drop your shoulders, and reach behind you, interlocking your fingers. Exhale into the stretch, keeping the chest lifted and shoulders down.

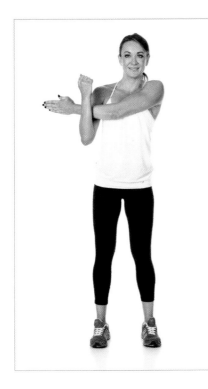

shoulder stretch

Put one arm across the body at shoulder height and hold it in place using the crook of your other elbow. Gently pull the straight arm toward you. Watch that your shoulder doesn't creep up—try to keep it down—and keep your neck long. Repeat on the opposite side.

triceps stretch

Bend one arm and put it behind your head. Using the other arm, hold the elbow and gently assist the stretch down. Keep the chest lifted and repeat on the opposite side.

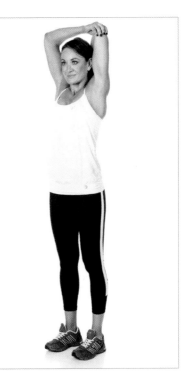

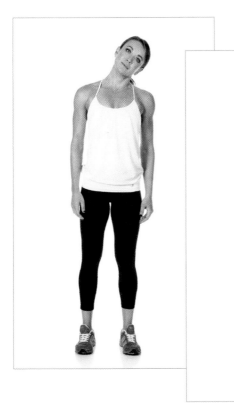

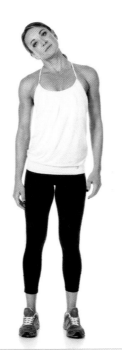

neck stretch

Lift your chest and drop your shoulders down away from your ears. Very gently lower your head to one side (ear to shoulder). Repeat on the opposite side.

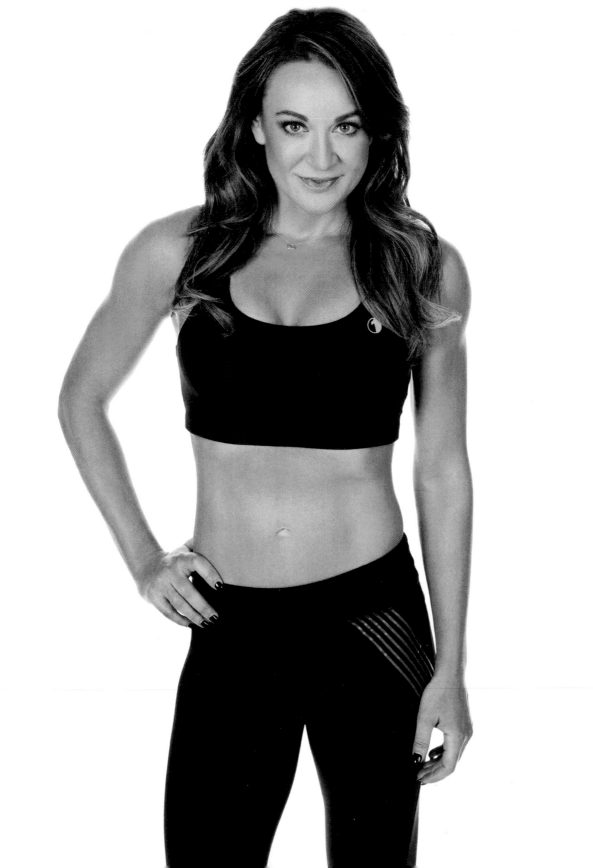

9
12-week new you routine

"if you miss a day, do not panic! get back on the horse; consistency is the key!"

Now it's time to combine the exercises you learned in the previous chapter to build a workout program that will deliver a killer result. You'll probably find yourself referring back to the exercises frequently for the first week or so, but after that they'll become second nature.

For dramatic results, you must follow these workouts (along with the nutrition plan in "Let's Get Cooking!"). It may seem daunting at first, especially if regular exercise is a whole new experience for you, but *I know you can do it!* I've trained hundreds of clients using these exercises, *and they work!* Having

said that, I want you to be flexible. If you can't get to the gym, or someone's taken over the spare room, then jog, run, jump rope, or cycle instead. As long as you're huffing and puffing, you're burning calories.

Each week will feature three days of fitness (cardio) training, two days of toning (weight) training, and one day of core strength. On your fitness day you can either do the circuit I've designed or choose one of the professional fitness classes I suggest. Most of the circuits will take you about 50 minutes, depending on how organized and focused you are. Most classes run for 50 minutes.

fitness days

- A fitness circuit is a series of exercises (20 repetitions each) performed one after the other without any rests in between. In my workouts you must go twice through the whole circuit. Closer to the end of the twelve weeks you'll do the circuit *three* times.

- You can set up the circuits either in the gym, the group fitness room, or even outside, as most of them use minimal equipment. However, you must check out your training schedule *before* your allotted exercise time, so you know exactly what you'll be doing and what you'll need.

- I've made Saturday a cardio training day, as most of my clients choose this day for their "treat meal." This way you can smash up the calories before you indulge.

toning days

- On toning days you can either choose a class like BodyPump or do the weights program I've devised for you.

- Where possible, you need to do your weights in super sets. This is where you do two different exercises, one for the upper body and one for the lower (15 repetitions each), and repeat the pair two or three times through. This will keep your heart rate up and in doing so burn tons of calories. Super sets can be tricky if your gym is busy, however, so be flexible—if it's not possible to use two pieces of equipment at once, simply stay with one exercise for 15 reps, have 45 seconds' rest, and then go again for another 15 reps before moving on to the next exercise.

- For the first two weeks the weights should be light: 2–5 pounds for your upper body and 10–15 pounds for your lower body,

rough guide to dumbbell weights (lbs)

| | female | | male | |
	upper body	lower body	upper body	lower body
Light	2–10	10–15	12–20	25–35
Medium	10–20	15–25	20–45	35–45
Heavy	20–45	25–45	45+	45+

depending on your gender and the exercise (see the "Rough Guide to Dumbbell Weights"). You must, however, increase your weights every two to three weeks to get the best results. How much you increase your weights will depend on the exercise and your fitness, but you should be really heaving by the last rep.

warm-ups

- There is also a warm-up for every training session. You *must* try to get your heart rate up to 140–150 bpm by the end of the warm-up.
- If you're not using a gym, simply replace any treadmill, elliptical trainer, or rowing machine warm-up with jogging or running (see pages 113–115 for running tips). Any "final blasts" that use the same equipment can be substituted with a lap around the block or park—whatever gets your heart rate up.

stretch

Do the stretch sequence on pages 127–131 at the end of every workout. Note, however, that if you do a BodyBalance, Pilates, yoga, or core class for your Friday workout, you won't need to do the stretch sequence that day.

If you miss a day, *do not panic*! Get back on the horse. Don't beat yourself up and use it as an excuse to throw in the towel. Consistency is the key! Good luck, and train *hard*!

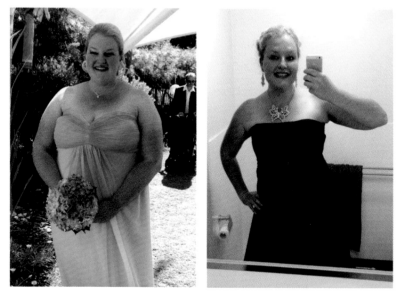

Kate
No excuses . . . train hard, eat clean, and watch your body transform.

michelle's seven-day workout diary

My exercise schedule changes regularly, depending on what I am training for and how many other commitments I have. Sometimes I focus more on weight training, at other times on classes or on running. I adore classes because they allow me to switch off and the music is great. Boxing is also *fantastic*! I have enlisted a boxing coach and he absolutely wrecks me!

When you read this diary, you need to remember that I am a *professional* trainer and that keeping fit is part of my job, so I have a pretty intense exercise routine. Plus I have to appear on national TV in Lycra! But it doesn't give you the excuse to say, "Oh, it's okay for her!" It's still hard for me and requires commitment and sweat, so you've got to get out there and do your bit. I usually break up my training into morning and afternoon sessions, though that also depends on my work commitments.

Monday	a.m.	Run 6.2 miles (52 minutes)	596 calories
	p.m.	BodyPump class (45 minutes)	410 calories
Tuesday	a.m.	Basic Training Circuit (50 minutes)	580 calories
	p.m.	Treadmill 6.2 mph (15 minutes)	148 calories
Wednesday	a.m.	Run 7.5 miles (60 minutes)	712 calories
	p.m.	Weights session (30 minutes)	278 calories
Thursday	a.m.	Boxing session (50 minutes)	758 calories
	p.m.	Indoor cycle class (45 minutes)	468 calories
Friday	a.m.	Run 7.5 miles (62 minutes)	736 calories
Saturday	a.m.	BodyPump class (45 minutes)	419 calories
	p.m.	BodyAttack class (45 minutes)	502 calories
Sunday		Rest	

"back-to-back classes—eek!"

week 1

This week is about getting your body used to exercise and equipment. On your fitness days, if you choose the circuit, remember to do each exercise 20 times, and the whole set twice. On your toning days, you'll do 15 repetitions of each exercise in the super set pair, but you must do each pair twice through before moving on to the next pair. Try to spike your heart rate above 140 bpm several times during your workouts. Perform 20 repetitions of the ab exercises twice through (two sets) on all days.

Remember—do all circuits with *urgency*!

monday:	fitness
WARM-UP	Treadmill 5 mins (3 mph, 2% incline)
CLASS	Indoor Cycle, Step *or*
CIRCUIT	

- Fast low-step running, right leg (p. 117)
- Fast low-step running, left leg (p. 117)
- Push-ups on knees (p. 93)
- Freestanding body-weight squat (p. 79)
- Standing shoulder press with light barbell or dumbbells (p. 96)
- Static lunge with support, 20 each leg (p. 81)
- Standing biceps curl with light barbell (p. 97)

ABS
- Crunches (p. 99)
- Leg extenion with right twisting crunch (p. 104)
- Leg extension with left twisting crunch (p. 104)

STRETCH

"on your toning days, remember to do each pair of exercises (super set) twice through before moving on to the next pair."

tuesday: toning

WARM-UP   Elliptical trainer 5 mins

CLASS   Strength training *or*

WEIGHTS
- Bent-over fly (p. 87) + Sumo squat with barbell (p. 86)
- Chest press with barbell (p. 90) + Exercise ball squat (p. 80)
- Towel pulls (p. 88) + Static lunge with support, alternating legs (p. 81)

FINAL BLAST   Treadmill 5 mins (3.5 mph, 2% incline)

ABS
- Crunches (p. 99)
- Leg extension with twisting crunch (p. 104), alternating left and right
- Plank on knees (p. 106), 30 secs

STRETCH

wednesday: fitness

WARM-UP   Treadmill 5 mins (3 mph, 2% incline)

CLASS   Boxing, Indoor Cycle, Step *or*

CIRCUIT
- Ski jumps (p. 122)
- Push-ups on knees (p. 93)
- Standing biceps curl with barbell (p. 97)
- Fast low-step running, right leg (p. 117)
- Fast low-step running, left leg (p. 117)
- Sprints (4 × 50 ft/15 m)
- Standing shoulder press with dumbbells (p. 96)

FINAL BLAST   Treadmill 5 mins (3.5 mph, 2% incline)

ABS
- Reverse crunch (p. 102)
- Leg extensions (p. 103)
- Lower body twist (p. 105)

STRETCH

thursday: toning

WARM-UP Rowing machine 5 mins

CLASS Strength training *or*

WEIGHTS

- Chest press with dumbbells (p. 91) + Sumo squat with barbell (p. 86)
- Bent-over fly (p. 87) + Step-ups with dumbbells (p. 84)
- Standing shoulder press with barbell (p. 96) + Exercise ball hamstring curl (p. 85)

FINAL BLAST Elliptical 5 mins

ABS
- Exercise ball crunch (p. 101)
- Exercise ball crunch with right twist (p. 101)
- Exercise ball crunch with left twist (p. 101)

STRETCH

friday: light fitness, core strength, and stretch

WARM-UP Cycle 15 mins (aim for 150+ bpm heart rate by end)

CLASS Pilates, Yoga, Core *or*

CIRCUIT

- Kneeling core and balance (right arm and left leg, holding last for 1 minute) (p. 108)
- Kneeling core and balance (left arm and right leg, holding last for 1 minute) (p. 108)
- Alternating back extension (p. 109)
- Leg extension with left twisting crunch (p. 104)
- Leg extension with right twisting crunch (p. 104)
- Lower body twist (p. 105)
- Leg extensions (p. 103)
- Reverse crunch (p. 102)

STRETCH Hold each for 2 mins—omit if you do a class

WARM-UP Treadmill 10 mins (3 mph, 2% incline)

CLASS Aerobics, Indoor Cycle, Step *or*

CIRCUIT

- Jump rope 1 min (p. 118)
- Backward power lunge, alternating legs (p. 82)
- Ski jumps (p. 122)
- Standing biceps curl with barbell (p. 97)
- Basketball jumps (p. 124)
- Standing shoulder press with light dumbbells (p. 96)

FINAL BLAST Treadmill 5 mins (3.5 mph, 2% incline)

ABS

- Leg extension with right twisting crunch (p. 104)
- Leg extension with left twisting crunch (p. 104)
- Lower body twist (p. 105)

STRETCH

"watch out for ski jumps and basketball jumps—these can be tough when you're just starting out, so start small and build up."

week 2

Now you're getting it! Remember that if you're not doing classes, you need to do 20 reps of each exercise in the fitness circuits, 15 of each in the weights workouts, and 20 of the ab exercises, all sets twice through. Try to spike your heart rate above 140 bpm several times during your workouts.

monday:	fitness
WARM-UP	Treadmill 5 mins (3 mph, 2% incline)
CLASS	Boxing, Indoor Cycle, Step *or*
CIRCUIT	

- Jump rope 1 min (p. 118)
- Push-ups on knees (p. 93)
- Basketball jumps (p. 124)
- Triceps bench dips (p. 98)
- Backward power lunge, 20 each leg (p. 82)
- Standing shoulder press with dumbbells (p. 96)
- Sprints (4 × 50 ft/15 m)

FINAL BLAST Treadmill 5 mins (3.5 mph, 2% incline)

ABS
- Plank on knees or toes 30 secs to 1 min (p. 106)
- Exercise ball crunch (p. 101)
- Exercise ball crunch with twist (p. 101)

STRETCH

tuesday: **toning**

WARM-UP Elliptical trainer 5 mins (3 mph, 2% incline)

CLASS Strength training *or*

WEIGHTS

- Towel pulls (p. 88) + Barbell squat (p. 79)
- Push-ups on toes to maximum, then finish on knees (pp. 94 and 93) + Backward power lunge, alternating legs, with light dumbbells (p. 82)
- Dumbbell rows, 15 each arm (p. 89) + Exercise ball squat with dumbbells (p. 80)

FINAL BLAST Treadmill 5 mins (3.5 mph, 2% incline)

ABS
- Lower body twist (p. 105)
- Leg extensions (p. 103)
- Crunches (p. 99)

STRETCH

wednesday: **fitness**

WARM-UP Jump rope 3 mins, cycle 3 mins (aim for 150+ bpm heart rate by end)

CLASS Boxing, Indoor Cycle, Step *or*

CIRCUIT

- Sprints (4 × 50 ft/15 m)
- Standing biceps curl with barbell (p. 97)
- Ice skaters on the spot (p. 121)
- Triceps bench dips (p. 98)
- Forward power lunge, alternating legs (p. 82)
- Ski jumps (p. 122)

FINAL BLAST Treadmill 5 mins (3.5 mph, 2% incline)

ABS
- Leg extensions with twisting crunch (p. 104)
- Reverse crunch (p. 102)
- Leg extension with twisting crunch, alternating right and left (p. 104)

STRETCH

thursday: toning

WARM-UP   Elliptical trainer 5 mins (using the handles)

CLASS   Strength training *or*

WEIGHTS

- Bent-over fly (p. 87) + Sumo squat with barbell (p. 86)
- Chest press with dumbbells (p. 91) + Static lunge with dumbbells, 15 each leg (p. 81)
- Standing shoulder press with dumbbells (p. 96) + Exercise ball hamstring curl (p. 85)

FINAL BLAST   Treadmill 5 min (3.5 mph, 2% incline)

ABS

- Supported crunch (p. 100)
- Supported crunch with medicine ball (p. 100)
- Supported crunch with twist (p. 100)

STRETCH

friday: light fitness, core strength, and stretch

WARM-UP   Cycle 15 mins or treadmill 15 mins (3.5 mph, 2% incline)

CLASS   Pilates, Yoga, Core *or*

CIRCUIT

- Alternating back extension (p. 109)
- Airplanes (p. 111)
- Lower body twist (p. 105)
- Plank on knees (30 secs) (p. 106)
- Leg extension with twisting crunch, alternating legs (p. 104)
- Kneeling core and balance (right arm, left leg, hold last for 1 min) (p. 108)
- Kneeling core and balance (left arm, right leg, hold last for 1 min) (p. 108)

STRETCH   Hold each for 2 mins—omit if you do a class

"in your weights workouts, don't forget to do each pair twice through before moving on to the next."

WARM-UP	Rowing machine 2 mins, plus 500 m (one-third of a mile) sprint
CLASS	Aerobics, Indoor Cycle, Step *or*
CIRCUIT	

- Sideways running, 3 steps each way (p. 119)
- Standing biceps curl with barbell (p. 97)
- Ice skaters on the spot (p. 121)
- Barbell squat (p. 79)
- Jump rope 1 min (p. 118)
- Standing shoulder press with barbell (p. 96)

FINAL BLAST	Treadmill 5 mins (3.5–3.7 mph, 2% incline)
ABS	

- Exercise ball crunch (p. 101)
- Exercise ball crunch with twist (p. 101)
- Kneeling core and balance, 20 each side (p. 108)

STRETCH

"push-ups on toes are hard, but brilliant for core strength—try just doing three or four, and even if they aren't very deep, it's a start!"

weeks 3 and 4

Now the intensity shifts up a gear. Increase your weights by 2–10 pounds in your weights workouts so that you're groaning by the last couple of reps. Sets and repetitions remain the same. Note that you'll be doing the same exercises for *two* weeks, which should help you get more familiar with them. Class-goers should have a go at doing the abs exercises *as well as* the occasional final blast.

monday:	fitness
WARM-UP	Treadmill 5 mins (3–4 mph, 4% incline)
CLASS	Indoor Cycle, Boxing, or Step *or*
CIRCUIT	
EXTRA WARM-UP	Treadmill interval jogs (no incline): 5 × 30 secs at 4–5 mph with 30 secs recovery
	• Push-ups on toes (p. 94) to your max, then finish on knees (p. 93)
	• Forward and backward jumps (p. 120)
	• Triceps bench dips (p. 98)
	• Sideways running, 3 steps each way (p. 119)
	• Standing shoulder press with barbell (p. 96)
	• Jumping jacks (p. 123)
FINAL BLAST	Cycle 5 mins (aim for 150+ bpm heart rate by end)
ABS	• Plank on knees (30 secs) (p. 106)
	• Exercise ball crunch (p. 101)
	• Exercise ball crunch with twist (p. 101)
STRETCH	

tuesday: toning

WARM-UP Elliptical trainer with handles 5 mins

CLASS Strength training *or*

WEIGHTS

- Towel pulls (p. 88) + Exercise ball squat with dumbbells (p. 80)
- Chest press with dumbbells (p. 91) + Static lunge (p. 81)
- Bent-over fly (p. 87) + Forward power lunge with dumbbells (p. 82)

FINAL BLAST Treadmill 5 mins (4–5 mph, 2% incline)

ABS
- Side plank (right 30 secs) (p. 107)
- Side plank (left 30 secs) (p. 107)
- Planks on toes (30 secs) (p. 106)

STRETCH

wednesday: fitness

WARM-UP Rowing machine 2 mins, plus 2 × 500-m rowing sprints (4 mins rest) (record your time)

CLASS Boxing, Indoor Cycle, Step *or*

CIRCUIT

- Walking push-ups on knees with one hand elevated (p. 95)
- Basketball jumps (p. 124)
- Triceps bench dips (p. 98)
- Jumping rope 1 min (p. 118)
- Ski jumps (p. 122)
- Sprints (4 × 50 ft/15 m)

FINAL BLAST Treadmill 5 mins (4–5 mph, 2% incline)

ABS
- Leg extensions (p. 103)
- Lower body twist (p. 105)
- Reverse crunch (p. 102)

STRETCH

thursday: toning

WARM-UP   Treadmill 5 mins (4–4.5 mph, 2% incline)

CLASS   Strength training *or*

WEIGHTS

- Towel pulls (p. 88) + Step-ups with dumbbells (p. 84)
- Chest press with barbell (p. 90) + Sumo squat with barbell (p. 86)
- Bent-over fly (p. 87) + Dynamic lunge with light dumbbells (p. 83)

FINAL BLAST   Treadmill 5 mins (4–5 mph, 2% incline)

ABS
- Crunches (p. 99)
- Reverse crunch (p. 102)
- Double crunch (p. 102)

STRETCH

friday: light fitness, core strength, and stretch

WARM-UP   Cycle 15 mins or treadmill 15 mins (3.5–4.5 mph, 2% incline)

CLASS   Pilates, Yoga, Core *or*

CIRCUIT

- Exercise ball back extension, alternating right and left (p. 110)
- Supported back extension on exercise ball (p. 112)
- Exercise ball crunch with right twist (p. 101)
- Exercise ball crunch with left twist (p. 101)
- Leg extension with twisting crunch (p. 104)
- Lower body twist (p. 105)

FINAL BLAST   Treadmill 5 mins (3 mph, 2% incline)

STRETCH   Hold each for 2 mins—omit if you do a class

"non-gym-goers, get more creative with your warm-ups: do a flight of stairs ten times, or run two blocks."

WARM-UP	Jump rope 5 mins, plus cycle 5 mins
CLASS	Aerobics, Indoor Cycle, Step *or*
CIRCUIT	
EXTRA WARM-UP	Treadmill interval sprints (incline level 1): 5 × 30 secs at 5.5–6.5 mph with 30 secs recovery

- Fast low-step running, right leg (p. 117)
- Fast low-step running, left leg (p. 117)
- Standing biceps curl with barbell (p. 97)
- Forward and backward jumps (p. 120)
- Push-ups on toes to your maximum, then finish on knees (p. 94)
- Ice skaters on the spot (p. 121)
- Sideways running, 5 steps each way (p. 119)

FINAL BLAST	Treadmill 5 mins (4–5 mph, 2% incline)

ABS
- Leg extension with right twisting crunch (p. 104)
- Leg extension with left twisting crunch (p. 104)
- Lower body twist (p. 105)

STRETCH

"if i've underestimated your fitness here and you can do more, go for it—don't hold back!"

weeks 5 and 6

Congratulations! You have one month under your belt, so now it's time to turn up the heat! Perform the super sets in the toning workouts *three* times through (still for 15 repetitions each) and try to spike your heart rate to 150 bpm several times each session. Stick to 20 repetitions for the fitness and abs exercises, but do them *three* times through (except for your 100-crunch ab days—Monday and Saturday). Once again, class-goers should do the abs, *plus* all the final blasts this time.

monday:	fitness
WARM-UP	Rowing machine 3 mins, plus a 500-m (one-third of a mile) sprint (record your time)
CLASS	Boxing, Indoor Cycle, Step *or*
CIRCUIT	
EXTRA WARM-UP	Treadmill interval sprints: 5 × 30 secs at 4–6 mph with 30 secs recovery
	● Forward and backward jumps (p. 120)
	● Standing shoulder press with barbell (p. 96)
	● Jump rope 1 min (p. 118)
	● Dynamic lunge, right (p. 83)
	● Dynamic lunge, left (p. 83)
	● Push-ups on toes to your max, then finish on knees (pp. 94 and 93)
	● Ice skaters on the spot (p. 121)
FINAL BLAST	Treadmill 5 mins (3.5 mph, 5% incline)
ABS	● Crunches × 100 (*one* set only) (p. 99)
STRETCH	

tuesday: toning

WARM-UP Elliptical trainer with handles 5 mins

CLASS Strength training *or*

WEIGHTS

- Bent-over fly (p. 87) + Sumo squat with barbell (p. 86)
- Chest press with dumbbells on exercise ball (p. 92) + Barbell squat (p. 79)
- Dumbbell rows (p. 89) + Dynamic lunge with dumbbells, 15 each leg (p. 83)

FINAL BLAST Treadmill 5 mins (4–5 mph, 2% incline)

ABS
- Leg extension with twisting crunch, alternating right and left (p. 104)
- Plank on knees then toes, 30 secs to 1 min (p. 106)
- Reverse crunch (p. 102)

STRETCH

wednesday: fitness

WARM-UP Treadmill 5 mins (3 mph, 6% incline)

CLASS Boxing, Indoor Cycle, Step *or*

CIRCUIT
- Triceps bench dips (p. 98)
- Ice skaters on the spot (p. 121)
- Basketball jumps (p. 124)
- Fast low-step running, right leg (p. 117)
- Fast low-step running, left leg (p. 117)
- Standing shoulder press with barbell (p. 96)
- Ski jumps (p. 122)

FINAL BLAST Treadmill 5 mins (4–5 mph, 2% incline)

ABS
- Leg extensions (p. 103)
- Lower body twist (p. 105)
- Side plank, knees or feet, 30 secs each side (p. 107)

STRETCH

thursday: toning

WARM-UP Jump rope 5 mins

CLASS Strength training *or*

WEIGHTS

- Chest press with barbell (incline bench) (p. 90) + Step-ups with dumbbells (p. 84)
- Towel pulls (p. 88) + Exercise ball squat with dumbbells (p. 80)
- Push-ups on toes (p. 94) + Barbell squats (p. 79) with 5 × 5 secs bottom halves (p. 78)

FINAL BLAST Treadmill 5 mins (3.5 mph, 6% incline)

ABS

- Leg extension with twisting crunch (p. 104)
- Supported crunch with medicine ball (p. 100)
- Planks on knees or toes 30 secs to 1 min (p. 106)

STRETCH

friday: light fitness, core strength, and stretch

WARM-UP Cycle 15 mins or treadmill 15 mins (3.5–4.5 mph, 2% incline)

CLASS Pilates, Yoga, Core *or*

CIRCUIT

- Kneeling core and balance (right arm, left leg, holding last one for 1 min) (p. 108)
- Kneeling core and balance (left arm, right leg, holding last one for 1 min) (p. 108)
- Kneeling core and balance, with diagonal reach, alternating (p. 108)
- Exercise ball crunch with twist, alternating right and left (p. 101)
- Exercise ball crunch with medicine ball (p. 101)
- Exercise ball alternating back extension (p. 110)
- Leg extension (p. 103)

FINAL BLAST Treadmill 5 mins (3.5 mph, 2% incline)

STRETCH Hold each for 2 mins—omit if you do a class

WARM-UP	Treadmill 5 mins (4.5 mph, 2% incline)
CLASS	Boxing, Indoor Cycle, BodyAttack, Step *or*
CIRCUIT	
EXTRA WARM-UP	Treadmill interval sprints: 10 × 30 secs at 5–6 mph with 30 secs recovery

- Walking push-up with one hand elevated (p. 95)
- Forward and backward jumps (p. 120)
- Sprints (4 × 50 ft/15 m)
- Sideways running, 3 steps each way (p. 119)
- Standing biceps curls (p. 97)
- Jumping jacks (p. 123)

FINAL BLAST	Treadmill 5 mins (3 mph, 7% incline)
ABS	• Exercise ball crunch × 100, *one* set only—try not to stop!
STRETCH	

"for dynamic lunges use a mirror, if you can,
to check your technique—as always, start with small steps
and build up to larger, faster ones and go slowly
when you use the dumbbells for the first time."

weeks 7 and 8

You should be pretty fit by now, and the fitter you are the harder you can work, so *go for it*! Aim to spike your heart rate at 150+ several times in the workouts. This week do your fitness circuit only *twice* through (I have added new drills to the beginning) except on Saturday, when you'll do it three times. For weights sessions stick to *three* sets of 15 reps, but you *must* be struggling by the last couple of reps. If you're not puffing, then increase the weight! Do your abs three times through (still 20 reps each). Once again, class-goers do the blasts and abs, too.

monday:	fitness

WARM-UP	Elliptical trainer with handles 5 mins
CLASS	Boxing, Indoor Cycle, Step, Aerobics *or*
CIRCUIT	
EXTRA WARM-UP	Treadmill interval sprints: 10 × 30 secs at 5–6 mph with 30 secs recovery

- Push-ups on toes (p. 94)
- Jumping jacks (p. 123)
- Standing shoulder press with barbell (light) (p. 96)
- Sideways running, 3 steps each way (p. 119)
- Basketball jumps (p. 124)
- Ski jumps (p. 122)

FINAL BLAST	Treadmill 5 mins (4–5 mph, 3% incline)

ABS
- Leg extension with right twisting crunch (p. 104)
- Leg extension with left twisting crunch (p. 104)
- Planks on knees or toes 1 min (p. 106)

STRETCH

tuesday: toning

WARM-UP Rowing machine 5 mins

CLASS Strength training *or*

WEIGHTS
- Double crunch (p. 102)
- Side plank, knees or feet, 30 secs each side (p. 107)
- Chest press with barbell (p. 90) + Sumo squat with barbell (p. 86)
- Bent-over fly (p. 87) + Step-ups with medium dumbbells, 15 right and 15 left (p. 84)
- Walking push-ups with one hand elevated (p. 95) + Exercise ball hamstring curl (p. 85)

FINAL BLAST Treadmill 5 mins (5–6 mph, 2% incline)

ABS
- Leg extensions (p. 103)

STRETCH

wednesday: fitness

WARM-UP Treadmill 5 mins (5–6 mph, 2% incline)

CLASS Boxing, Indoor Cycle, Step *or*

CIRCUIT

EXTRA WARM-UP Treadmill jog 15 mins (4.5 mph, 2% incline) or walk 15 mins 3 mph, 12% incline)
- Forward and backward jumps (p. 120)
- Ice skaters on the spot (p. 121)
- Triceps bench dips (feet elevated) (p. 98)
- Jump rope 1 min (p. 118)
- Backward power lunge, alternating legs (p. 82)
- Sprints (6 × 50 ft/15 m)

FINAL BLAST Rowing machine 500 m sprint (record your time)

ABS
- Supported crunch with medicine ball (p. 100)
- Leg extensions with twisting crunch (p. 104)
- Lower body twist (p. 105)

STRETCH

thursday: **toning**

WARM-UP Elliptical trainer 5 mins

CLASS Strength training *or*

WEIGHTS
- Towel pulls (p. 88) + Exercise ball squat with dumbbells (p. 80)
- Chest press with dumbbells on exercise ball (p. 92) + Static lunge with medium barbell, 15 each leg (p. 81)
- Dumbbell rows, 15 each arm (p. 89) + Sumo squat with barbell (p. 86)

FINAL BLAST Treadmill 5 mins (5–6 mph, 2% incline)

ABS
- Reverse crunch (p. 102)
- Exercise ball crunch (p. 101)
- Exercise ball crunch with twist, alternating right and left (p. 101)

STRETCH

friday: **light fitness, core strength, and stretch**

WARM-UP Cycle 15 mins or treadmill 15 mins (3.5–4 mph, 2% incline)

CLASS Pilates, Yoga, Core *or*

CIRCUIT
- Kneeling core and balance (right arm, left leg, holding last one for 1 min) (p. 108)
- Kneeling core and balance (left arm, right leg, holding last one for 1 min) (p.108)
- Kneeling core and balance, with diagonal reach, alternating (p. 108)
- Side plank, 1 min each on right and left (p. 107)
- Leg extension with twisting crunch, alternating right and left (p. 104)
- Planks on knees or toes, 1 min (p. 106)
- Leg extensions (p. 103)
- Reverse crunch (p. 102)

FINAL BLAST Treadmill 5 mins (3.5–4 mph, 2% incline)

STRETCH Hold each for 2 mins—omit if you do a class

WARM-UP	Treadmill 5 mins (5–6 mph, 2% incline)
CLASS	Boxing, Indoor Cycle, Step *or*
CIRCUIT	
EXTRA WARM-UP	Treadmill interval sprints: 10 × 30 secs at 5–6 mph with 30 secs recovery

- Walking push-ups with one hand elevated (p. 95) + Sprints (4 × 50 ft/15 m)
- Dynamic lunge right (p. 83) + Sprints (4 × 50 ft/15 m)
- Dynamic lunge left (p. 83) + Sprints (4 × 50 ft/15 m)
- Standing biceps curl with barbell (p. 97) + Sprints (4 × 50 ft/15 m)
- Ice skaters on the spot (p. 121) + Sprints (4 × 50 ft/15 m)
- Triceps bench dips (p. 98) + Sprints (4 × 50 ft/15 m)
- Take a 3-min breather then go again, twice more

FINAL BLAST	Elliptical trainer 5 mins
STRETCH	

"there are no abs on saturday because I want you to
do the circuit three times."

weeks 9 and 10

By now, some of you may have already reached your target weight, especially if your plan was to lose 10–20 pounds. For those who still have more to lose, seek and destroy! The new fitter, stronger, healthier, sexier you must do *three* sets of 20 reps in your circuits and abs and *three* sets of 15 reps in your weights workouts. Your target is to spike your heart rate to 150+ bpm several times. As usual, repeat these exercises for two weeks, and class-goers do blasts and abs.

monday:	fitness
WARM-UP	Elliptical trainer 5 mins
CLASS	Boxing, Indoor Cycle, Step, Aerobics *or*
CIRCUIT	

- Jump rope 1 min (p. 118) + Sprints (4 × 50 ft/15 m)
- Shoulder press (p. 96) + Sprints (4 × 50 ft/15 m)
- Basketball jumps (p. 124) + Sprints (4 × 50 ft/15 m)
- Triceps bench dips (p. 98) + Sprints (4 × 50 ft/15 m)
- Squat jumps (p. 79) + Sprints (4 × 50 ft/15 m)
- Take a 2-min breather then go again, twice more

FINAL BLAST Treadmill 5 mins (4 mph, 6% incline)

ABS
- Crunches × 150 (p. 99)

STRETCH

tuesday: toning

WARM-UP Elliptical trainer with handles 5 mins

CLASS Strength training *or*

WEIGHTS

- Towel pulls (p. 88) + Step-ups (high bench) with dumbbells, 15 each leg (p. 84)
- Chest press with dumbbells (p. 91) + Barbell squat (p. 79)
- Dumbbell rows, 15 each arm (p. 89) + Exercise ball hamstring curl (p. 85)

FINAL BLAST Treadmill 5 mins (5–6 mph, 2% incline)

ABS
- Leg extension with right twisting crunch (p. 104)
- Leg extension with left twisting crunch (p. 104)
- Reverse crunch (p. 102)

STRETCH

wednesday: fitness

WARM-UP Rowing machine 3 mins, plus 500-m (one-third of a mile) sprint (record your time)

CLASS Aerobics, Boxing, Indoor Cycle, Step *or*

CIRCUIT

EXTRA WARM-UP Treadmill jog 20 mins (5–6 mph, 2% incline), or 10 mins at 5–6 mph (2% incline) *plus* 10 mins at 3.5 mph (12% incline)

- Walking push-ups with one hand elevated (p. 95)
- Forward and backward jumps (p. 120)
- Standing shoulder press with barbell (p. 96)
- Ice skaters on the spot (p. 121)
- Backward power lunge, 20 each leg (p. 82)
- Sideways running, 5 steps each way (p. 119)

FINAL BLAST Cycle 5 mins

ABS
- Supported crunch with medicine ball (p. 100)
- Supported crunch with medicine ball with twist (p. 100)
- Supported crunch (no ball) (p. 100)

STRETCH

thursday:	**toning**

WARM-UP Elliptical trainer 5 mins

CLASS Strength training *or*

WEIGHTS

- Chest press with dumbbells on exercise ball (p. 92) + Exercise ball squat with dumbbells, narrow stance (p. 80)
- Dumbbell rows (p. 89) + Forward power lunge with dumbbells, 15 each leg (p. 82)
- Standing shoulder press with dumbbells (p. 96) + Leg press (p. 86)

FINAL BLAST Treadmill 5 mins (5–6 mph, 2% incline)

ABS
- Leg extension with twisting crunch, alternating right and left (p. 104)
- Planks on toes 1 min (p. 106)
- Exercise ball crunch (p. 101)

STRETCH

friday:	**light fitness, core strength, and stretch**

WARM-UP Cycle 15 mins (aim for 150+ bpm heart rate by end)

CLASS Pilates, Yoga, Core *or*

CIRCUIT

- Leg extension with twist (p. 104)
- Plank on knees or toes (hold for one 1 min) (p. 106)
- Alternating back extension (p. 109)
- Airplanes (p. 99)
- Crunches × 10 with 10-sec hold at top (p. 99)
- Reverse crunches × 10 with 5-sec hold at top (p. 102)

FINAL BLAST Treadmill 5 mins (3.5 mph, 2% incline)

STRETCH Hold each for 2 mins—omit if you do a class

*"because you should really know your exercises by now,
I don't give you page references to look them up."*

WARM-UP Jump rope 5 mins

CLASS Running, Aerobics, Boxing, Indoor Cycle, Step *or*

CIRCUIT

- Push-ups on toes (p. 94) + Sprints (4 × 50 ft/15 m)
- Sideways running, 3 steps each way (p. 119) + Sprints (4 × 50 ft/15 m)
- Triceps bench dips, feet elevated (p. 98) + Sprints (4 × 50 ft/15 m)
- Forward and backward jumps (p. 120) + Sprints (4 × 50 ft/15 m)
- Standing biceps curl with barbell (p. 97) + Sprints (4 × 50 ft/15 m)
- Forward power lunge, alternating legs (p. 159) + Sprints (4 × 50 ft/15 m)
- Take a 1-min breather then go again, twice more

FINAL BLAST Treadmill 10 mins (3.5 mph, 6% incline)

ABS
- Exercise ball crunch (p. 101)
- Exercise ball crunch with right twist (p. 101)
- Exercise ball crunch with left twist (p. 101)
- Lower body twist (p. 105)

STRETCH

weeks 11 and 12

This is it. It's been a long time in the making, but you've arrived at the final workouts! On your fitness days, do *three* sets of 20 reps, and on your toning days, do *three* sets of 15 reps, but keep increasing the weights so that your last couple of reps are real groaners! For your abs, do *three* sets of 20 reps. Your heart rate should be high enough so that you are breathless for most of the workout. Beat your best times in *all* your warm-ups! Class-goers do warm-ups, abs, *and* final blasts. This is the *home stretch*—get mad, get mean, get macho!

monday:	fitness
WARM-UP	Rowing machine 3 mins, plus 500-m (one-third of a mile) sprint
CLASS	Boxing, Indoor Cycle, Step *or*
CIRCUIT	
	● Push-ups on toes (p. 94) + Sprints (4 × 50 ft/15 m)
	● Dynamic lunge (right) (p. 83) + Sprints (6 × 50 ft/15 m)
	● Dynamic lunge (left) (p. 83) + Sprints (8 × 50 ft/15 m)
	● Shoulder press with barbell (p. 96) + Sprints (10 × 50 ft/15 m)
	● Take a 2-min breather then go again, twice more
FINAL BLAST	Elliptical trainer 5 mins
ABS	● Crunches × 200 (I mean it—break them into sets of 20 reps if it helps) (p. 99)
	● Jump rope 1 min (p. 118) + Sprints (4 × 50 ft/15 m)
STRETCH	

tuesday: toning

WARM-UP Treadmill 5 mins (5–6 mph, 2% incline)

CLASS Strength training *or*

WEIGHTS

- Towel pulls (p. 88) + Step-ups with dumbbells (p. 84)
- Chest press with dumbbells (heavy) (p. 84) + Exercise ball hamstring curl (p. 85)
- Dumbbell row, 15 each arm (p. 89) + Forward power lunge with dumbbells, 15 each leg (p. 82)

FINAL BLAST Cycle 5 mins (aim for 150+ bpm heart rate by the end)

ABS
- Leg extensions with twisting crunch (p. 104)
- Crunch with right twist holding medicine ball (p. 101)
- Crunch with left twist holding medicine ball (p. 101)
- Reverse crunch (p. 102)

STRETCH

wednesday: fitness

WARM-UP Elliptical trainer 5 mins, plus rowing machine 500-m sprint *(beat your time!)*

CLASS Boxing, Indoor Cycle, Step *or*

CIRCUIT

EXTRA WARM-UP Treadmill interval sprints: 10 × 30 secs at 5–7.5 mph with 30 secs recovery
- Forward and backward jumps (p. 120)
- Triceps bench dips (p. 98)
- Over-the-fence jumps (p. 124)
- Push-ups on toes (p. 94)
- Basketball jumps (p. 124)
- Ice skaters on the spot (p. 121)

FINAL BLAST Treadmill 5 mins (5–6 mph)

ABS
- Double crunch (p. 102)
- Lower body twist (p. 105)
- Leg extensions (p. 103)

STRETCH

thursday:	**toning**

WARM-UP	Treadmill 5 mins (5–6 mph)
CLASS	Strength training *or*
WEIGHTS	

- Towel pulls (p. 88) + Exercise ball squat with dumbbells (heavy) with 5 × 8 bottom halves (p. 80)
- Dumbbell rows (p. 89) + Dynamic lunge with medium dumbbells, 15 each leg (p. 83)
- Chest press with barbell, flat bench (p. 90) + Squat with barbell (p. 86)

FINAL BLAST	Rowing machine 5 mins
ABS	

- Leg extensions (p. 103) + Crunch with twist, alternating right and left (p. 104)
- Planks on toes 1 min (p. 106)
- Exercise ball crunch with medicine ball (p. 101)

STRETCH

friday:	**light fitness, core strength, and stretch**

WARM-UP	Cycle 15 mins (aim for 150+ bpm heart rate by end)
CLASS	Pilates, Yoga, Core *or*
CIRCUIT	

- Exercise ball alternating back extension (p. 110)
- Hand knees or toes (hold for 1 min) (p. 106)
- Alternating back extension (p. 109)
- Airplanes (p. 111)
- Crunches × 10 with 10-sec pause at the top (p. 99)
- Reverse crunches × 10 with 5-sec pause at top (p. 102)

FINAL BLAST	Treadmill 5 mins (3.5 mph, 2% incline)
STRETCH	Hold each for 2 mins—omit if you do a class

"over-the-fence jumps are tough, but you'll easily have enough strength for these now."

WARM-UP	Jump rope 5 mins
CLASS	Aerobics, Boxing, Indoor Cycle, Step *or*
CIRCUIT	

- Ski jumps (p. 122)
- Walking push-ups with one hand elevated (p. 95)
- Ice skaters on the spot (p. 121)
- Push-ups on toes (p. 94)
- Over-the-fence jumps (p. 124)
- Sideways running, 5 steps each way (p. 119)
- Sprints (8 × 50 ft/15 m)

FINAL BLAST	Treadmill 5 mins (3 mph, 15% incline)
ABS	• Exercise ball crunch × 150
STRETCH	

"do today's circuit four times through, just because you can!"

what now?

Congratulations! You have done what so many can only dream of. You have completed a full three months of training. I have no doubt that some days were harder than others and that you experienced the good, the bad, and the downright ugly! But you are here, you survived, and now you know what you are capable of—far more than you ever thought, right?

So let's talk weight. How much have you lost? And how much more do you have to lose? For those of you who have nailed your goal weight, no doubt you are feeling invincible! Some of you may have even shifted the goal posts—many of my clients do when they get to this point. Instead of aiming for a size 10, they are now eyeing a size 8. That's brilliant, and I encourage you to go for it. It may mean repeating another few weeks of workouts, but by now you will be a savvy exerciser, and you'll know how long and how hard you need to go to burn the calories.

For those of you who are out to drop 100 or more pounds, you should be at or just past your halfway mark. My guideline for you is crystal clear: you will do the full twelve weeks of workouts again, obviously upping the intensity to match and challenge your current fitness. I know you can do it—the weight you have already lost is proof of that. Remember that contestants on *The Biggest Loser* train for sixteen weeks, and they have me yelling at them all day long. If you're out to lose more than 100 pounds, six months is a realistic timeline.

This is where you do not drop the ball and leave the game. That may have been where you took a wrong turn last time, but remember, you are doing things differently this time.

Whether you are at your goal weight or at the halfway point, there are a few things that will never change:

- You are an exerciser. It's who you are—you brush your teeth, you make your bed, you train. You will do an hour's exercise six days a week and look forward to it because you know how fantastic it makes you feel. You will always take the stairs instead of the elevator and walk instead of taking the car because you know that every bit of informal exercise helps—and because it just feels right.
- You are careful with what you eat. You will always make the smart choices, you will always know where you are with your calorie intake, and you will keep workin' that kitchen to become a great low-calorie chef!
- You set yourself up for success by *choosing* to train hard and eat well every day.

This is what you will do. And the reward? A happier, healthier, sexier you! One hundred percent worth it!

"this is where you do not drop the ball and leave the game—remember, you are doing things differently this time."

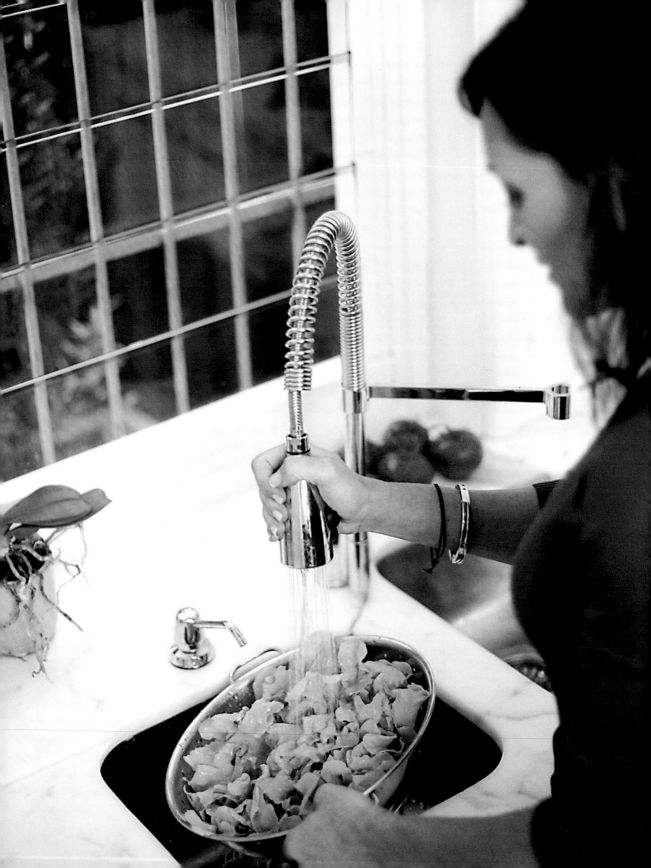

let's get cooking!

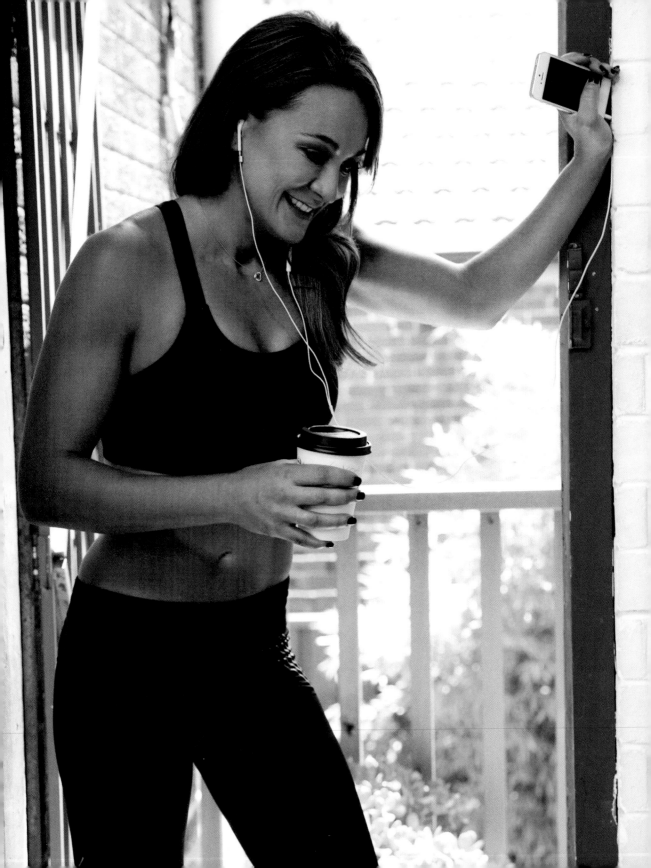

10
nutrition

"losing weight always comes down to what you put in your mouth—end of story!"

Chances are that if you are overweight, you are food-obsessed. You may even be addicted to food. Tough call, I know, but check in with yourself. How much of your day do you spend eating? Add to this the time you spend preparing food or getting yourself to places where you can buy or eat food. Then add the time that you are thinking and talking about food. If you've got quite a few hours totaled up, then clearly you have an *emotional* relationship to food.

An emotional relationship to food is a consistent pattern with overeaters. If you find yourself turning to food when you're stressed or unhappy, or if eating huge quantities of calorie-dense junk is something you associate with reward, celebration, and good times, then you've moved away from the principle

of food for sustenance. Food for you has come to mean something different.

There's nothing new about using food as a celebration. We've been doing it for centuries, when special occasions were marked by feasting that sometimes went on for days. The difference is that in the modern age, this "celebration" food is available *every day* and *everywhere*. Nowadays, it doesn't have to be a special occasion for us to partake in a five-course meal—any day that ends in a *-y* will do just fine!

junk food

Readily available junk food and our ever-increasing desire to eat it have resulted in an explosion of fast-food outlets, rocketing us to

> *"let me tell you, there are entire shopping aisles you must never visit again if you are to reach your goal."*

the number one position on the global obesity charts. Compare our eating habits to those of other Western countries, and then compare the availability of calorie-dense takeout outlets and you'll see why France, Italy, or any other country that has resisted the influx doesn't have the same obesity issues that we have.

Because fast-food manufacturers work in huge volumes, their products are cheaper—it's no coincidence that obesity is more prevalent in less-affluent areas. Yet we've *all* been fooled into thinking that it's actually cheaper to eat fast food than whole food. It isn't. We've also been brainwashed to believe that it's more convenient, which we sometimes use as an excuse to make poor food choices: "I haven't got time to cook. I'll just grab some takeout." I guarantee you can make a healthy, nutritious meal in less than 20 minutes, and that it costs a quarter of the price.

Yet fast food is not the only junk food. Let's take a walk around your average supermarket and see what else qualifies, starting with the first meal of the day—breakfast. Around 80 percent of breakfast cereals can be classified as junk, despite claims for added vitamins, as they generally include loads of added sugar. And let's not forget sodium (salt). Did you know that there is a cereal marketed to children that has more sodium per serving than a bag of chips?

My classification of junk food also includes all those ready-made pies and other dishes in the frozen-food section, and the entire cakes and cookies section. Add to the list soft drinks, sugary juices, and all the potato chips and snacks that are cleverly located next to them. It includes most of the ready-made sauces and packages of just-add-water slop. Ditto the entire candy section, most of the canned fruits, dips, white breads, margarine, and all those "snacks in a box."

Don't get sucked in by the "low-fat" label, either. If it's low-fat, then the nutritional label should prove it to you beyond doubt. Low-fat foods can still be high in calories if they contain a lot of sugars (carbohydrates). The quickest way to check their suitability is to check the label for the calorie content—but *beware*! When you look at the number of calories *per serving*, make sure that the serving size is the amount you would normally eat, and not some paltry offering.

The biggest problem, however, with a lot of these low-fat, low-calorie foods is that they're often low in nutritional value as well and, being ready-made, prevent you from learning about food preparation. Don't let the food companies dumb you down! Let me tell you, there are *entire shopping aisles* you must *never* visit again if you are to reach your goal.

If that sounds scary, hear this, because it may well be the most important thing you'll read. While exercise will do *amazing* things for your mind, your body, and your spirit, losing weight will always come down to what you put in your mouth! *End of story!*

If I had two clients, one of whom refused to eat well and ate whatever she liked whenever she liked, but I trained her like a demon every day, and another who did no exercise but tidied up her diet so that she had a weekly calorie deficit, the non-exerciser would lose the most weight.

Of course the best scenario is the double-whammy approach:

- Good nutrition + exercise = FAST RESULTS!
- Fast results = BETTER MOTIVATION!
- Better motivation = EVEN FASTER RESULTS!

what's really in your food?

Now, I'm no chemist, but a little bit of science helps to explain why food does what it does, and why some foods lead us to needing a separate zip code for our butts while others don't.

We have four major sources of energy: protein, carbohydrates, fats, and alcohol. Yes, alcohol. You need to understand the role of *all* the energy sources you put into your body, and although, strictly speaking, alcohol is just another carbohydrate (it's not even a food by definition, because it doesn't supply any micronutrients, such as vitamins and minerals), it's one that is omnipresent in the modern era and is totally relevant in the weight loss debate.

You need to understand the distinction between calorie-dense and nutrient-dense foods. Nutrient-dense foods generally contain fewer calories, so we can eat more of them. These are what we call whole foods, and they include unprocessed meat, poultry, fish, fruit, vegetables, and grains that have been refined as little as possible (such as in whole-grain bread). Be aware, though, that not all whole foods are low in calories, which is why you can *still* be overweight with a healthy diet. A great example of this is an avocado, which is a whopping 500 calories!

food type	calories per gram
Carbohydrates (fruit, vegetables, grains)	3.8
Protein (nuts, eggs, chicken, beef, etc.)	4.0
Fat (oil, butter, milk, cheese)	8.8
Alcohol	6.4

Calorie-dense foods generally have fewer nutrients and are often higher in fat or sugar, or both. At the top end are chips, ice cream, chocolate, burgers, hot dogs, etc., most containing the nutritional value of a sock.

carbohydrates

Carbohydrates would have to be one of the most contentious, confusing, and overanalyzed foods. This is all you need to understand:

- Carbohydrates are found in most foods.
- Our bodies use carbohydrates to make glucose, which gives us energy and allows our brains to function properly.
- Because our bodies use *all* carbs for fuel, it's up to us to choose ones that are high in nutrients and low in calories—that is, whole foods.

low-GI carbohydrates

The GI (glycemic index) is a measure of how fast carbohydrates enter the bloodstream. Low GI is rated at 55 or less, medium GI is 56–69, and high GI is 70 or more. High-GI foods are not necessarily bad, in fact they are fantastic if you are about to run a race and need a quick hit of energy. However, diabetics and weight loss candidates should stick to low- and occasionally medium-GI foods. It's no coincidence that unrefined whole foods are generally low GI.

carbohydrate-rich whole foods

Brown rice
Fruit and vegetables
Honey
Milk
Minimally processed cereals (bran, muesli, oats)
Rice noodles
Whole-grain pasta and bread

protein

Protein is essential for the building and repair of all body tissue, including muscles, skin, blood, hair, and organs. Protein is found in meat, fish, dairy products, seeds, nuts, and legumes. It makes you feel full, which can prevent overeating, and it's really easy to dish out the right portion size (a chicken breast half, a palm-sized piece of steak). Just make sure you remove all the fat.

protein-rich whole foods

Lean red meats (beef, lamb)

Lean poultry (chicken, turkey)

Fish and shellfish

Eggs

Milk, cheese, yogurt

Tofu

Legumes (beans, peas, chickpeas, lentils, peanuts)

Nuts and seeds (walnuts, almonds, pumpkin seeds, sunflower seeds)

fats

Fats or fatty acids are an important energy source and are required for healthy skin and some body functions. Fats should make up around 20–30 percent of our daily calorie intake, but we need to be careful to eat the right kind of fats.

protein shakes

Protein shakes are an excellent supplement if you are training hard because they assist with muscle recovery. I use them to increase my protein levels if I don't feel like eating meat for every meal or if I'm in a rush to get to work. They're also great if I am about to go out for a really late dinner and need to put something in my tummy (it means I'm less likely to pig out at dinner, too). Protein shakes can also be very useful for vegetarians.

All fats are high in calories. Watch out for nuts in particular. While they are nutritious, they're also calorie-dense. Dieticians recommend eating only ten almonds as a snack, but who stops at ten? I never recommend them for snacks—they're just too tempting. I'd rather use them in my cooking or scatter them in a salad, because that way I eat less; likewise with avocados and olive oil. When it comes to storing calories, your body does not differentiate between good and bad fats.

alcohol

Only your liver can metabolize alcohol, and while it's busy doing that, any excess alcohol

the good guys

Monounsaturated fats are easily used as fuel and help decrease cholesterol levels.	Foods high in monounsaturated fats include olive oil, canola oil, peanut oil, avocado, almonds, peanuts, cashews, macadamias, hazelnuts, pecans, and eggs.
Polyunsaturated fats (found in oily fish and plant foods) include omega-3 and omega-6 fats, which are essential fatty acids (they're crucial to our health but our bodies can't make them). Omega-3 fats have been shown to help prevent heart disease.	Foods high in omega-6 fats: eggs, cereals, poultry, pine nuts, seeds, vegetable oil (sunflower, safflower, soybean, corn). Foods high in omega-3 fats: salmon, sardines, tuna, mackerel, anchovies, trout, herring, flaxseed oil, walnuts, eggs.

the bad guys

Trans fats (also called hydrogenated fats) are polyunsaturated fats that have been treated so they remain solid at room temperature. They're used extensively in foods (always check the label) and are crap.	You'll often see them in commercial chips, pastries, doughnuts, cookies, muffins, cakes, pies, and margarine.
Saturated fats (found in meat and dairy products) are more readily stored as body fat than unsaturated fats and are less easily used as fuel. They also raise blood cholesterol levels.	Common sources of saturated fats include meat fat, chicken fat, butter, full-fat milk/yogurt, cream, cheese, coconut milk, palm oil, and deep-fried fast food.

floats around in your bloodstream messing up other organs (like your brain). Your body breaks down foods *preferentially*, and it will always metabolize alcohol first, then carbohydrates, followed by fats and, as a last resort, protein. This sounds okay, until you remember that last night you were chowing down on potato wedges with sour cream and cashew nuts while you slurped a few beers! And then you went and had dinner with a few more drinks to boot! Your body will be using the alcohol to fuel itself before it uses the food, so guess where all that food will go? Storage, anyone?

The other thing with alcohol, of course, is that when we drink we tend to make dumb food choices that can ruin days of careful exercise and nutrition. Alcohol is *evil* for weight loss.

get organized

I cannot overstate the impact of your diet on your weight. Food occupies a much larger part of your life than exercise ever will. Work it out—you train for an hour, six days a week. That's six hours. You'll spend a significant percentage of the other 162 hours organizing yourself for, preparing, being tempted by, or eating food. So always be guided by the number one rule: what goes into your mouth will make the most difference.

To start eating right you need to surround yourself with high-quality whole foods and be well organized in the kitchen. This means your kitchen will need a significant makeover and you'll need to say goodbye to some old friends. You know the ones: the chocolate sauces, the boxes of cookies (just in case you have visitors—yeah, sure, girlfriend!), the dumb breakfast cereals, the cans of soda.

Here's what to do. Go outside and get your big trash can. Wheel it into your kitchen and put it in the middle of the room with the lid open. Starting at the pantry and working your way around the entire kitchen, grab any unhealthy crap and launch it *straight into the trash can.* As you do, shout, "Get the hell out of my life—I'm *over* you holding me back!"

If you have to stop and think about a particular item for more than 5 seconds, then throw it away anyway, for wasting your time. If you sample any of them, then please give yourself a slap across the face from me! And no, don't give me the old "But it's such a waste . . ." Let me tell you what a waste is. A waste is having spent the last ten or twenty years of your life with a weight issue that has been hanging around your neck and dragging you down, down, down. A waste is missing out on the fabulous life that is rightfully yours! You deserve more, more, more!

Next, take a trip to the supermarket and restock your fridge, freezer, and pantry with the good stuff. I've made shopping lists for you in the next chapter. This way you'll beat your instincts at their own game by surrounding yourself with food that'll make you *slim*, not food that'll make you *fat*. You are taking control now.

cook the right stuff

Just as you are now an exerciser, you are now a cook. There is no way on this planet that you can accelerate yourself to lean and mean unless you put in some time in the kitchen. Not only is cooking easy, it also makes you take responsibility for your own nutrition, and that is an important step toward taking responsibility for your own body. And if you have children, you'll know that this will be one of the best gifts you can give them. This is a long-term gift, not a short-term quick fix. And you can even get them involved in the cooking process.

My approach to cooking is to keep it simple, and you'll notice that the recipes in Chapter 13 reflect just that. I don't think too many of us have time during the week to prepare gourmet meals, so the recipes are quick and simple with a minimum of ingredients. For some, I've also included a fancier variation that you might want to try on the weekend, or when you've got more time to spend in the kitchen. It's a good idea to occasionally cook more than you need so that you have a couple of extra servings to freeze or have for lunch the next day.

vegetables and fruit

And now for the ingredients. When you open the fridge or pantry door, you want to be faced with fresh vegetables such as zucchini, carrots, and sweet potatoes. You want to see asparagus, tomatoes, broccoli, and onions. You want to be able to dive into an ocean of apples, kiwi fruit, bananas, and passion fruit. You want to immerse yourself in an abundance of grapes, melon, and mango, and when you do, you should rub it all over you, inhale it, and sink into it, groaning in

"there is no way on this planet that you can accelerate yourself to lean and mean unless you put in some time in the kitchen."

john's heartwarming story

In the third season of Australia's *The Biggest Loser* we had an older man named John who came into the house with a severe heart condition, so severe that his cardiologist banned him from doing any exercise apart from walking for a maximum of 30 minutes three times a day, and even then he wasn't allowed to let his heart rate go above 100 beats per minute (about 57 percent of his maximum heart rate). He was put on a strict whole-foods diet and he walked for half an hour three times a day. After the first ten days John had lost over 20 pounds! He went on to lose more weight and got fitter, and he was eventually given clearance to do any exercise he wished! Truly one of the most incredible turnarounds I've ever witnessed.

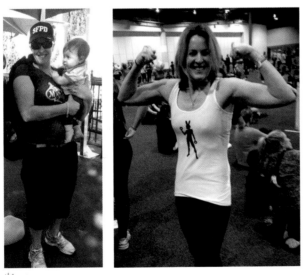

Katie
Lost 50 pounds

"I love this program. It's helped me achieve my dreams and beat postpartum depression."

orgasmic rapture, because *this is the stuff that will keep you alive.* The other stuff is slowly poisoning you.

You think I'm exaggerating? Let me ask you a question. When you've gone back for your second helping of cheesecake, how do you feel afterward? Bloated? A bit sick? You betcha! That's because your body is trying to reject it. It knows that the cheesecake is poisonous to the wonderful molecules and other particles that make up your amazing body, the one that you *love*. Remember?

meat

In the Western world, our diet is largely meat-based. Ask your co-workers what they had for dinner the night before and most of them will usually start with "beef" or "chicken." Historically, meat was the food of the wealthy, so it was something of a treat. Now it is comparatively cheap and it's everywhere—quite a lot of it attached to our guts, actually.

Your new diet is *not* going to be meat-based—it's going to be vegetable-based. In countries where meat is difficult to come by because of price or availability, it makes up a much smaller part of the average meal— think Southeast Asia and the like. And it's no coincidence that these countries generally don't have too many XXXLs roaming around.

So your new approach to meat is to use it almost as a garnish—much smaller portions, around 5 to 7 ounces, but well prepared with yummy homemade marinades or spicy toppings.

Of course, the big plus is that vegetables are low in calories, so you can eat lots and lots of them without putting yourself into calorie surplus. How do five asparagus spears, two carrots, a large floret of broccoli, a cup of spinach, and a couple slices of yellow squash sound? Enough to complement your marinated chicken breast? That's a pretty hefty plate of vegetables, but it's only 120 calories.

control your portions

Most people are overweight because they ingest too many calories, too much food— more food than their bodies actually need. Sure, there can be issues around hormones, prescription drugs, and the like, but for the most part people simply *eat too much.*

Take a long, hard look at your portions. There's a good chance you are eating twice as much as you need. You may have been eating hefty portions for so long that you don't even realize *how* big they are. Yes, cutting them is going to be a little uncomfortable at first. You've trained your stomach to expect *way* more than it needs, so it's probably going to let you know how it feels about the new portions. But you won't die! You will still be able to fill your belly and keep the hunger at bay, but it will be with nutrient-dense, low-calorie whole foods rather than those with zero nutrients and a gazillion calories.

Here are some smart rules to help you reduce portions:

- Use smaller plates.
- Never go back for seconds. They never taste as good, and you don't need them.
- Never finish off anyone else's food.
- Never eat while you are cooking.

Remember the 7-Day Food Diary I asked you to keep in Chapter 4? This should have given you a handle on the amount of food you are eating. To work out the calories, you would have needed to weigh food and read the labels on cans and boxes. Now, before you start worrying about having to measure and weigh your portions for the rest of your life, don't panic. All I'm asking is that you keep a detailed food diary while you're doing your twelve-week training program. Although you may not keep a food diary forever, you will always keep a mental tally of your calo-

ries. Within the first week or so you'll know a reasonable-sized portion just by looking at it, but you'll need to check every couple of weeks that your portions haven't crept up.

Your portions will depend on your calorie quota per day, which in turn depends on your gender and weight (see page 40), but in general, use the following as a guide:

your daily calorie quotas

women

3 meals × 350 cals each
1–2 snacks × 150 cals each
Total = 1,350 cals

men

3 meals × 400 cals each
1–2 snacks × 200 cals each
Total = 1,600 cals

eat regularly

Stop playing games with yourself. You know the ones: "Well, I've hardly eaten all day, so now I can gorge myself" or "If I skip breakfast and only have an apple for lunch, then I can dive into a buffet and a case of beer." Before you know it, you'll have taken in more calo-

is it really "low-fat"?

Any smart city girl or boy knows that the way to get the best food on an airline, and to get it before everyone else, is to put yourself down for special dietary requirements. So naturally I've always insisted on a low-fat meal to keep my calorie count down. My long-time business partner and friend gets the everyday stuff, so on one particularly long flight we decided to kill some time with a calorie-count comparison of our meals.

We estimated that my "low-fat" meal (a banana, OJ, Special K, skim milk, and a berry bar) totaled around 552 calories with 9.6 grams of fat—without tea or coffee. Now, that's a pretty big breakfast (it was the "healthy" bar that blew it at 250 calories). I'd normally be shooting for 350 to 450 tops, so I chucked the bar and stayed within my limit.

Billy got his meal, cereal and toast complete with whole milk and butter, and it came in at 520 calories, 32 calories *less* than mine! The message? Unless you take responsibility for your own food, *you don't have a chance*. Calorie-dense food is everywhere, because it tastes good and the food companies know that. They've designed it to give your taste buds instant gratification when it makes contact— never mind that you feel like you've swallowed a brick afterward.

ries than if you'd eaten breakfast and lunch put together. So give up the games. They do not work, and they will leave you feeling tired and angry with yourself.

From now on you will eat breakfast, lunch, *and* dinner. You will have a snack during the day only if you need the energy, and you will no longer binge at night. Your focus will be on eating more during the day when you need it and less at night.

- Eat like a king for breakfast.
- Eat like a prince for lunch.
- Eat like a pauper for dinner.

Eat your evening meal as early as you can, brush your teeth, pull the plug, *game over*! Okay, I get that you have a life. Stuff comes up, like birthdays, events, and parties. I get it. However, it's what you do 95 percent of the time that counts. The *occasional* Saturday night here or there won't make a difference if you are keeping it clean the rest of the time.

forget low-fat!

Okay, here we go—deep breath. *If you want to lose weight quickly, forget low-fat.* (Collective gasp of horror from the entire Western world.) Let me qualify that just a little before the avalanche of hate mail arrives from the food companies. If your primary goal is to lose weight, your primary concern should be the *number of calories you eat*. Now, this doesn't mean you can eat crap provided you stay within your daily calorie count, because crap isn't nutritious and won't keep your body functioning properly. What it means is that when you're standing in the supermarket squinting at the nutrition label on the side of a container of yogurt, the first thing you should look at is the calorie content per serving. After that, check out the fats, sugars, and other components. The calorie content is inextricably linked to the fat content, anyway: more fat equals more calories.

We've been told for decades that we should buy "lite," "low-fat," or "fat-free." Now we're being told to buy "low-carb." At the end of the day, fat is *not* the most important factor in making your weight loss food choices. What have we got to show for twenty years of low-fat eating? The obesity epidemic. That's because even though the foods available to us are low in fat, they are still frequently high in calories, and our "inner Labrador retriever" has always read "low-fat" as "eat more" anyway. Once again, *know your calories.*

reduce alcohol intake

Speaking from experience, if there's one thing that kills your willpower, it's alcohol. Get a few drinks in you and suddenly all that inner strength goes down the toilet, often along with the booze. On top of that, alcohol is full of calories and is mostly consumed at night when you should be taking in fewer calories, not more. Then when you train the next day (and you *will* train with a hangover—you play, you pay) your body uses the alcohol first for energy, which sounds good on the face of it, until you remember that you didn't exactly reach for a fruit salad

"if your primary goal is to lose weight, then your primary concern should be the number of calories you eat."

last night, either. It was more like cheese, crackers, chips, dips, and, oh yeah, the pizza at 3:00 a.m. Limit alcohol to two nights a week and keep it in check. For faster results, cut it out completely.

snack right

As you learned in Chapter 8, your body will go into panic mode if you do not eat regularly, and will begin to store energy (fat) if it suspects there's a chance of starvation. Healthy snacks will prevent this, and will also stop you from making dumb food choices because you're too hungry to think straight. However, don't feel you have to snack between meals—if you're *really* not hungry, wait until your next meal.

be creative

The essence of tasty, nutritious food is variety and freshness. When you go to one of those very posh restaurants where the menu describes every ingredient in each dish, check out the range of products they use—sauces, spices, herbs, and seeds are all added to several fresh core ingredients to make the dish truly memorable.

But it isn't just the taste that is good. Variety also improves the nutritional value of the

healthy snacks

- 8-oz cup low-fat plain yogurt with a couple of strawberries (150 cals)
- 6 small rice crackers, each with ½ tablespoon low-fat cottage cheese (110 cals)
- 1 medium raw carrot dipped in 3 tablespoons low-fat ricotta (120 cals)
- 1 pint strawberries (115 cals)
- 4-oz basket blueberries (80 cals) (way cheaper than a coffee and a muffin, and so much better for you!)
- 3 sesame wheat crackers with vegetable spread (150 cals)
- 3 slices apple (½ inch thick) topped with 1 tablespoon low-fat ricotta and mint leaf (120 cals)
- 10 snow peas, 10 snap peas, and 10 green beans (50 cals)
- 2 celery sticks spread with 3 tablespoons low-fat ricotta (120 cals)

meal, and richly colored veggies are especially nutritious. So instead of sticking a frozen breaded fish fillet in a frying pan and serving it with mashed potatoes, try a fresh fish fillet marinated in lemon juice, ginger, garlic, scallions, and a drizzle of sesame oil. Wrap it in foil and stick *that* in the oven. Then steam some whole Brussels sprouts with florets of cauliflower and broccoli until they're tender, dust them with paprika and cracked pepper, and lightly toss them in a nonstick frying pan with a spray of extra-virgin olive oil. Both meals are basically fish and vegetables. One is crap and has the nutritional equivalent of soap. The other will make you feel good and let you live a long and slender life. One has three ingredients (if you include the bread crumbs). The other has twelve ingredients and doesn't taste like cardboard.

The same rule applies to all meals. Breakfast? Half a cup of rolled oats mixed with flaxseed, sliced almonds, raisins, chopped dates, sunflower seeds, and pumpkin seeds with skim milk, half a sliced banana, and a little bit of low-fat yogurt. Getting the picture?

Another reason to be creative with herbs and spices is that when you first start eating whole foods, your taste buds will tell you it's bland because they're used to loads of salt,

sugar, and artificial flavors. Don't worry, though. Your taste buds will come back to life—just as you will when you start eating good food.

be human

Each week I allow myself and my clients to have a treat meal, which includes all their favorite things. Shannan, my *Biggest Loser* colleague, calls them his "cheat meals." Often when we have been out together and a rather delicious-looking dessert turns up, he will say, "Mish, do ya think it's worth a cheat?" In other words, is this what we *really* want for our treat?

I usually set aside Saturday night for my treat meal. And to counterbalance that, I will train like a woman possessed on Saturday morning. This way I go into Saturday night really looking forward to having a delicious meal with dessert *and* alcohol, all guilt-free. Then Sunday I'm back on the healthy-life program. Remember, this is a single treat meal, not a treat day.

11
your kitchen makeover

"your kitchen is ground control in the war on weight loss!"

To set yourself up for success, you'll need to visit the supermarket or produce market at least once a week. Keep an ongoing shopping list stuck to the fridge door and add to it as you run out of fresh ingredients. When you have a bit more time on the weekend, try visiting local fresh food markets—it's much cheaper and you will always find new and interesting produce to experiment with.

Be smart when storing your vegetables in the fridge: it will make a big difference in how long they last. My mom gave me a great tip: if your breakfast cereal comes in a waxy plastic bag, reuse it to store your veggies. Fold down the top and seal with a clip and your veggies will last an entire week, sometimes longer!

Now, before I go any further, let me get this off my chest: I'm not a vegetarian but I *am* thoughtful about my food choices. I'll buy organic if I can, but it's not a deal breaker for me. I won't, however, buy cheap tomatoes that taste like water. Nor will I buy fluffy-textured apples that have obviously been on a slow boat from half a world away. I absolutely won't buy an egg or meat from a caged bird, and I don't buy endangered fish like red snapper, orange roughy, or swordfish—and that goes for when I'm eating out, too.

Note also that I don't do fruit juices because they are full of calories. If you like juice, get a juicer and do it yourself, but make sure you add it to your daily calorie tally.

If you are only cooking for one, don't go out and buy *everything* on the shopping lists below—just select what you think you might get through in a week. Also, some foods will be better (and cheaper) in season. It will take you a couple of weeks to find the balance of how much produce to buy so that you have minimal waste. Once you get the hang of it, cooking your favorite quick and easy meals will save you money, make your butt smaller, and teach you to appreciate food in a very different way.

fridge

- Asparagus (put into a glass of water and stand in the fridge to last longer)
- Carrots
- Eggplant
- Free-range eggs
- Fresh corn
- Fruit
- Garlic (fresh or in a jar)
- Ginger (fresh or in a jar; I usually freeze my fresh ginger and grate it frozen)
- Green veggies (broccoli, bok choy, kale, zucchini)
- Low-fat cottage cheese or ricotta cheese
- Low-fat (skim) milk (cow or soy)—high-calcium is best
- Low-fat yogurt, no sugar
- Meat for sandwiches (some people like to have lean deli meat like ham or turkey,

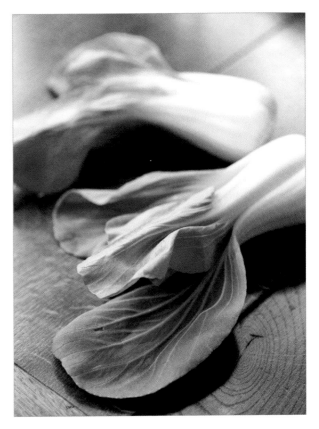

though I'm not a big fan, as these tend to be salty; another option is to cook an extra chicken breast when you're preparing a main meal, and to use that instead)
- Multigrain or soy and flaxseed bread
- Onions, leeks
- Parmesan (a strong-flavored cheese like this means you only need to use a little)
- Salad veggies (arugula, baby spinach, basil, cucumber, mushrooms, celery, peppers)

pantry

- Anchovies
- Canned beans (red kidney beans, chick-peas, butter beans, and others—be sure to rinse them before eating or cooking)
- Canned tomatoes
- Canned tuna, salmon, sardines
- Capers
- Chili sauce (use sparingly)
- Cold-pressed extra-virgin olive oil (you'll use less because it's strongly flavored)
- Couscous
- Dried beans (taste better and contain less sugar and salt than canned versions, but need to be soaked overnight)
- Dried pasta
- Fresh tomatoes (avoid refrigerating fresh tomatoes—they taste better at room temperature)
- Herbs and spices (mixed herbs, paprika, dried basil, oregano, cinnamon, cumin)
- Light soy sauce (use sparingly)
- Low-fat hot chocolate mix (make sure there are no trans fats)
- Low-GI cereal (e.g., Special K)
- Olive oil spray
- Olives
- Oyster sauce (look for MSG-free, though there's sugar and salt in this, so use sparingly)
- Pepper grinder full of black peppercorns

- Rice (brown)
- Rolled oats
- Seeds (sesame, pumpkin, sunflower)
- Sesame oil
- Stock (cartons or cubes—check the sodium content)
- Raisins
- Tomato paste
- Tomato-based sauces (no added sugar)
- Untoasted muesli
- Vinegar for dressings (balsamic, red wine)
- Whey protein powder

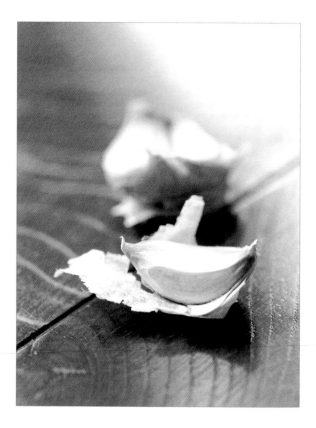

freezer

- Free-range, skinless chicken breasts
- Fish fillets (white-fleshed fish, salmon)
- Lean red meat (boneless beef)
- Frozen peas
- Frozen berries (blueberries or raspberries are better value frozen than fresh, last longer, and are yummy in oatmeal or yogurt)
- Multigrain or flaxseed bread

utensils

To get around the kitchen quickly, you'll need some decent utensils, and I've gotta tell you, I have a deep attachment to a lot of my kitchen bits and pieces because they let me do what I need to do when I need to do it. My must-haves include:

- A nonstick wok
- Two nonstick frying pans—one big, one small
- A good set of stainless-steel saucepans with a steamer basket
- A couple of cutting boards
- Chef's knife (these are the big suckers with a 6-to-8-inch blade; if you buy a cheap one you'll be sharpening it forever, so get the best you can afford)
- Paring knife
- Knife sharpener
- Silicone utensils (not nylon—it melts and is toxic)
- Kitchen scale
- Measuring cups and spoons
- Salad spinner
- Airtight containers for leftovers

the snowball theory

You know the cartoon where a snowball starts rolling down a mountain and gets bigger and bigger and faster and faster? That's what your metabolism is like once you get it up and running with regular exercise and good nutrition. When you have your one treat meal each week, it's a bit like a single tree standing up in the snow. When the snowball strikes, it takes the tree out, no problem, and just keeps on rolling. The snowball does have a problem, however, if that single tree becomes a forest. Are you hearin' me?

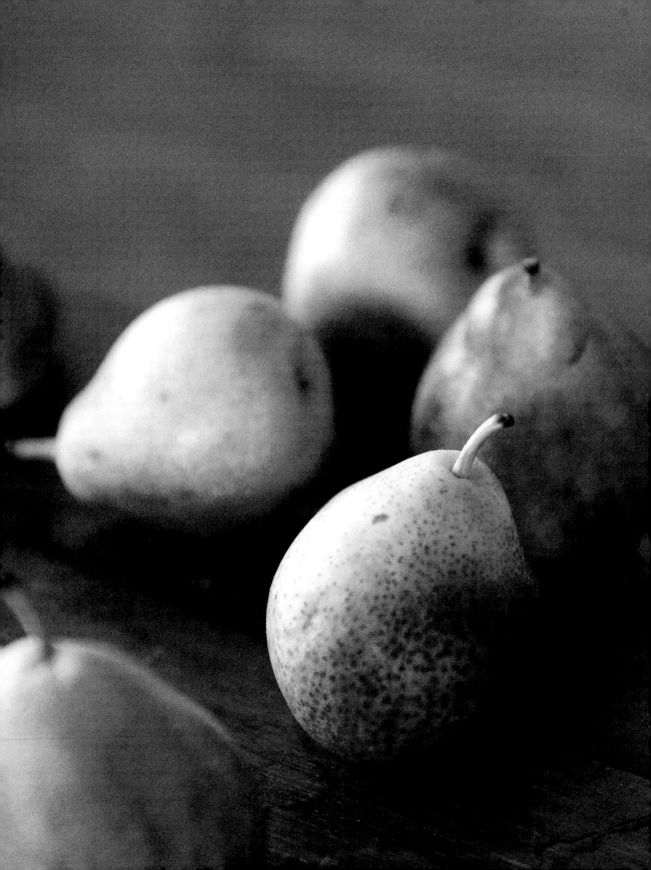

12

a simple eating plan

"now it's up to you to become a calorie commando!"

I put all my clients on a nutrition plan that features a specific calorie quota per day. The calorie quota will depend on their gender and weight, and it will usually *decrease* gradually as the pounds come off and their lighter bodies need less fuel for energy.

Most of my big male clients (350+ pounds) start on 1,800–1,900 calories per day, slowly reducing to 1,600 calories as they lose more weight. I usually put my heavy female clients (300+ pounds) on around 1,600 calories and get them down to about 1,300–1,400. For clients who have only 10–20 pounds to lose, I put the males on 1,400–1,600 calories and the females on 1,200–1,300. Factors such as exercise, hormones, and medication can alter these fig-

ures (speak to your doctor about this), but for most people, these are the formulas that work.

Personally, I keep my calories between 1,200 and 1,300 per day, which is light for someone who exercises as much as I do, but with the right food, I never go hungry. In order to stay full and satisfied I eat a lot of low-calorie foods, which is why there's plenty of salad, vegetables, fruit, and lean meat in my diet. My portions are not out of control, nor do I go back for seconds. If there are leftovers, I put them in a container for lunch the next day.

I eat throughout the day and I eat very well. The worst thing you can do is skip meals, as it will always come back to haunt you. You always end up feeling starved, and

how many calories?

One of my male clients weighed 385 pounds, was 5'11", and had a BMI of 52.87—in other words, morbidly obese. I started him at 1,800–1,900 calories per day, and as he lost weight, pulled him down to around 1,600 calories per day.

He was used to taking in around 4,200 calories daily, so instead of 29,400 calories per week, he was now consuming just 13,300 calories per week. We know that 2 pounds of body weight represent around 7,000 calories, so he was set to lose roughly 5 pounds a week without factoring in the training.

One of my female clients weighed 297 pounds, was 5'5", and had a BMI of 48.39—also morbidly obese. She was used to a daily calorie intake of around 2,700 calories, so I started her at 1,600 calories per day and gradually reduced that to 1,300–1,400 calories. Once we got her training, she actually lost 7 pounds in the first week!

it's usually at night—the worst time to take on loads of calories!

I try to stick to my rule of eating like a king for breakfast, a prince for lunch, and a pauper for dinner. Of course, it doesn't always work, especially on the weekends. But when I know I am going out for dinner I will keep my calories a bit lower during the day so I have some room to move during the evening and don't feel like I'm missing out.

I allow myself only one treat meal and one chocolate treat each week; even so, they really add up, especially if I have alcohol! No wonder people stack on the weight if they eat and drink like this more than once a week. On my treat-meal day I always pump up my training to compensate.

On pages 192–193 you'll find a sample eating plan for a female client wanting to lose 45 pounds in 12 weeks. But anyone can use it—simply adjust the daily calories to suit your own daily calorie intake goal. You heavy guys out there may need to beef up your breakfasts and lunches (*not* the dinners), increasing the portion sizes to get up to 1,800 calories per day. Be sure, though, to gradually decrease your daily intake as the weight starts to come off. I have calculated the calories for each meal, so you can mix and match the meals to get the right quota.

Now it's up to you to become a *calorie commando*! Choose low-calorie whole foods and fill yourself up on them. Memorize the calories of the foods you regularly eat so that you don't have to keep looking them up. Keep checking in on where you are on your calorie intake as the day progresses. When I'm working on *The Biggest Loser,* the first two questions I ask my team members are "How many calories have you burned?" and "How many calories have you eaten?" and they *always* know. They are making conscious and responsible choices—you can do it, too!

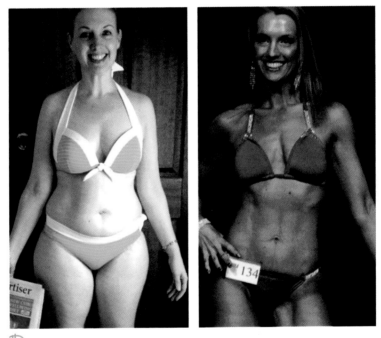

Dee
From flabby to fitness competitor!

	breakfast	cals	snack	cals
Day 1	Egg-White Omelette w/o toast (see p. 198)	70	1 medium apple	70
	1 pear, chopped	70		
	1 cup low-fat yogurt	80		
	1 coffee with skim milk	100		
	total	320	total	70
Day 2	½ cup oats, cooked with water	135	4 whole-grain crackers with	
	½ cup skim milk	45	hummus	115
	1 small banana, chopped or mashed	65		
	¼ cup frozen or fresh berries	60		
	total	305	total	115
Day 3	2 slices multigrain toast	180	1 medium banana	85
	2 tbsp cottage cheese	35	1 medium apple	70
	1 sliced tomato with pepper and		1 coffee with skim milk	100
	lemon juice	30		
	1 kiwi fruit	40		
	10 strawberries, sliced	30		
	total	315	total	255
Day 4	2 boiled eggs	140	2 whole-grain crackers	100
	2 slices toasted whole-grain bread	180	2 tbsp cottage cheese	60
	1 cup low-fat yogurt	80	½ pear, sliced	45
	total	400	total	205
Day 5	1 kiwi fruit	40	1 coffee with skim milk	100
	1 nectarine	25		
	1 peach	45		
	1 banana	65		
	15 grapes	30		
	10 strawberries	30		
	1 cup low-fat yogurt	80		
	total	315	total	100
Day 6	½ cup untoasted muesli	160	1 slice cinnamon raisin bread	100
	1 cup high-calcium skim milk	90	1 level tbsp low-fat ricotta cheese	30
	10 chopped strawberries	30	1 coffee with skim milk	100
	total	280	total	230
Day 7	2 slices toasted multi-grain bread	180	1 large banana	120
	2 heaping tbsp cottage cheese	60	1 coffee with skim milk	100
	1 cup mushrooms, grilled	20		
	1 onion, grilled	30		
	1 tomato, grilled	30		
	1 cup spinach, steamed	5		
	total	325	total	220

lunch	cals	snack	cals	dinner	cals	total cals
1 can tuna in spring water	200	2 whole-grain crackers	50	Stir-Fry with beef (see p. 205)	300	
1 medium mixed salad (arugula, basil, cucumber, peppers, strawberries, grapes)	60	2 tbsp cottage cheese	60			
1 slice whole-grain bread	90	1 large carrot	30			
total	350	total	140	total	300	1,180
5 oz lean chicken breast, grilled	230	1 cup fresh strawberries	30	5 oz salmon steak, grilled	300	
1 medium green leafy salad	60			1 cup mixed veggies (broccoli, squash, zucchini, spinach), steamed	50	
1 slice whole-grain bread	90			1 small ear corn	110	
total	380	total	30	total	460	1,290
2 salmon hand rolls (sushi	240	2 carrots	40	Chicken Drumsticks in Tomato Broth (see p. 208)	330	
1 small Greek salad	120	1 large celery stick	2			
total	360	total	42	total	330	1,302
Stir-Fry with chicken or beef (see p. 205)	300	1 peach	45	3½ oz boneless steak, grilled	180	
				2 cups mixed veggies (carrots, bok choy, mushrooms, peppers, eggplant), steamed	120	
total	300	total	45	total	300	1,250
Penne with Feta and Lemon (see p. 212)	480	2 Fig Newtons	110	Barbecued Kebabs (see p. 214)	360	
total	480	total	110	total	360	1,365
2 slices whole-grain bread	180	1 peach	45	Pan-Fried Shrimp and Scallops with Orange and Tomato (see p. 202)	260	
1 heaping tbsp cottage cheese	30	1 large apple	75			
3 slices lean ham	75	1 kiwi fruit	40			
½ tomato	15			1 cup hot chocolate (made with hot water)	60	
½ cup lettuce and grated carrot	20					
total	320	total	160	total	320	1,310
1 large multigrain roll	160	1 cup low-fat yogurt	80	1 Vegetarian Stack (see p. 211)	360	
3½ oz tuna	90					
½ cup salad	20					
total	270	total	80	total	360	1,255

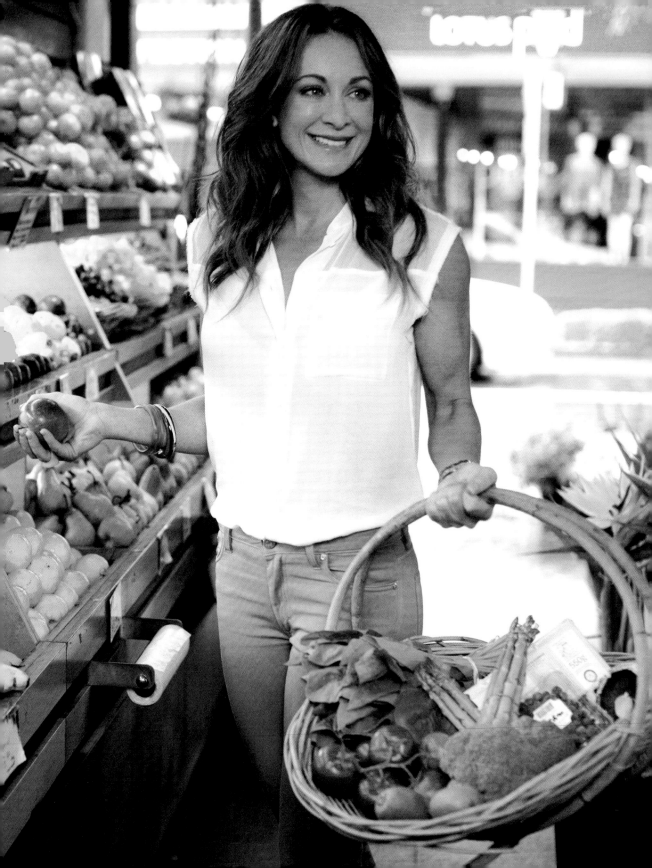

13
recipes

"I don't think too many of us have time during the week to channel our inner gordon ramsay, so my meals are quick and simple."

As I noted earlier, if you're a foodie and you've got plenty of time to spend in the kitchen, these recipes may not be for you. There are some great cookbooks out there that describe how to prepare delicious low-calorie foods, but for me, a lot of the recipes are just too time-consuming. The principle of my cooking is this: I follow simple recipes, usually with three to five ingredients, and I just add the herbs, spices, seeds, oils, nuts, and other bits and pieces as I feel like it. (I often base my choices around what I have left in the fridge or pantry.) During the week I simply don't have time to be pureeing twice-cooked white beans or

doing any other time-consuming food prep. That's why God gave us restaurants. I need my recipes to be quick, delicious, and right on my calorie count. On the weekends I might get a bit more adventurous, so I've suggested variations at the end of some of the recipes.

breakfast

These are my top breakfast recipes. Always buy high-protein whole-grain bread. You won't be eating that much bread anyway, so there's no point eating second-rate stuff.

cottage or ricotta cheese on toast

Use a good-quality whole-grain bread, and choose part-skim or low-fat cheese. If you don't have fresh herbs, used dried, though halve the quantity. Around 300 calories.

Serves 1

2 slices whole-grain bread, toasted
2 teaspoons chopped fresh mint or chives
1 small clove garlic, peeled and cut in half
½ cup low-fat ricotta or cottage cheese

While the bread is toasting, stir the mint or chives through the cheese. Rub the cut side of the garlic over the toast. Spread cheese mixture over the toast and serve while the toast is still warm.

egg-white omelette with toast

A big favorite of mine—high in protein, quick to prepare, and filling. All in all, about 220 calories per serving.

Serves 1

5 egg whites
1 scallion, chopped
Freshly ground black pepper
4 cherry tomatoes, halved
Olive oil spray
1 slice whole-grain bread, toasted
1 small clove garlic, peeled and cut in half

Whisk the egg whites in a bowl. Add the scallion (or sprinkle in some dried mixed herbs instead), pepper, and tomato. Heat a small nonstick frying pan and spray with olive oil. Pour in the egg mixture and cook for 2–3 minutes or until cooked through. Fold over and serve on a slice of toasted bread that has been rubbed with garlic.

Variation: Try adding ½ cup baby spinach or flat-leaf parsley and 3–4 sliced mushrooms to your egg whites. Alternatively, a dash of Tabasco or paprika will give it a kick, or add some fresh thyme or fennel. I love freshly ground fennel seeds—they're so aromatic! Alternatively, steam a handful of baby spinach, drizzle with lemon juice, sprinkle some sesame seeds on top, and serve on the side. You'll deserve it after you've destroyed yourself in the gym or beaten your best time on your Saturday-morning run!

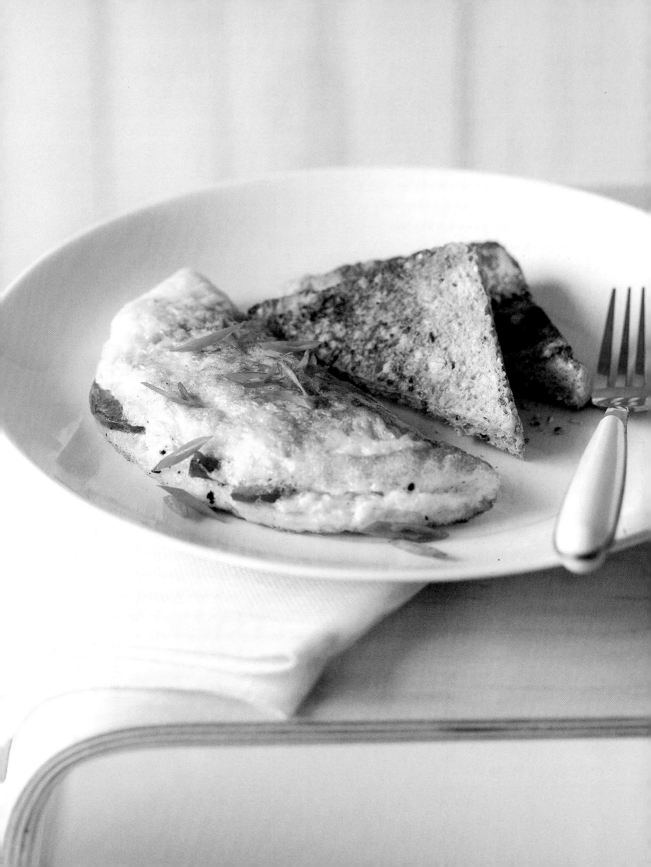

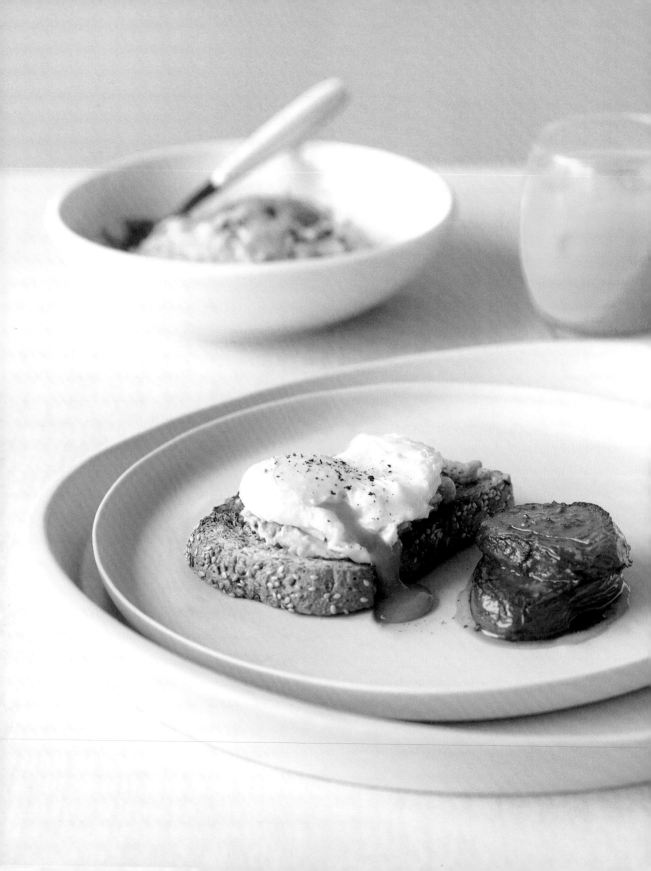

poached egg on toast

Especially good if you buy organic free-range eggs. All in, it's 250 calories.

Serves 1

1 tablespoon white vinegar
1 egg
1 tablespoon mashed avocado
1 slice whole-grain bread, toasted
Freshly ground black pepper

Half fill a small saucepan with water and add the vinegar. Bring almost to a boil, and just as the little bubbles are rising to the surface, reduce the heat a bit and stir the water vigorously to create a little whirlpool (don't scald yourself!). Carefully crack the egg on the side of the saucepan and release the contents into the middle of the whirlpool—this will stop the white from going all over the place. Fish it out with a slotted spoon after 2 minutes for a softer egg, or 3 minutes for a harder texture. Spread the avocado on a piece of toast and pop the egg on top. Add a bit of ground pepper and there you go! Be careful with the avocado, though—it's loaded with calories.

A simpler variation: If that all sounds a bit long-winded, then simply fry the egg in a pan sprayed with olive oil—the calories are almost the same. Squeeze some lemon juice on the avocado and garnish with chives and watercress, or add grilled tomato and mushrooms or steamed spinach on the side.

oatmeal

This is my all-time favorite winter breakfast. Make sure the ingredients label reads "oats"—nothing else. This breakfast is around 270 calories, including the raisins.

Serves 1

½ cup rolled oats
1 cup (250 ml) skim milk
1 heaping tablespoon raisins or a dollop of honey or brown sugar (optional)
Sprinkling of ground cinnamon (optional)

Place the oats and milk in a small saucepan. Bring to a boil, reduce the heat to low, and cook for 5 minutes, stirring occasionally. Stir in the raisins. If it's looking too thick and heavy, add water. If you don't like raisins, add a dollop of honey or brown sugar to sweeten. Sprinkle some cinnamon on top if you like.

Variation: To lower your calorie count, cook the oats in water, then add ¼ cup skim milk to serve. To beef it up, mash a banana and cook with the oatmeal (this will add 100 calories). Serve with a sprig of mint.

fruit and yogurt

This combination always reminds me of summer. Take the time to find a good-quality low-fat yogurt. Always use fresh fruit, never canned, as canned is full of sugar. Calorie count for this one is around 300.

Serves 1

1 cup low-fat yogurt
3 pieces fresh fruit (banana, kiwi fruit, pear), chopped
1 sprig of mint, chopped

Spoon yogurt into a bowl and place the fruit on top. Sprinkle with chopped mint to serve.

Variation: Add two of the following (these are listed in *ascending* order of calorie content): strawberries, blueberries, raspberries, fresh figs, blackberries, grapes, dates, sunflower seeds, raw almonds, raw cashews, and sesame seeds. (Keep an eye on those nuts and seeds—they have around *ten times* the calories of grapes!) Add a squeeze of lime juice for extra zing.

homemade muesli with yogurt

Prepare this on the weekend so it's ready for the following week. If making your own muesli is not your idea of fun, then grab a bag of untoasted muesli from the grocery store that fits your calorie target (it needs to be no more than 350 calories per 100 grams). Beware the ones with buckets of dried fruit, as they're super sweet and full of sulfur, though if the rest of it looks okay you could always pick out the suspect fruit.

Serves 4

2 cups rolled oats
½ cup bran
1/3 cup sunflower seeds
1/3 cup pumpkin seeds (pepitas)
2/3 cup chopped pitted dates
¼ cup raisins
1 cup skim milk or low-fat yogurt, or a mix of both

Combine all the ingredients except milk or yogurt and store in an airtight container. To serve, place half a cup of muesli in a bowl and add skim milk, low-fat yogurt, or both to serve.

Variation: Serve with strawberries or grapes—they're low in calories and delicious.

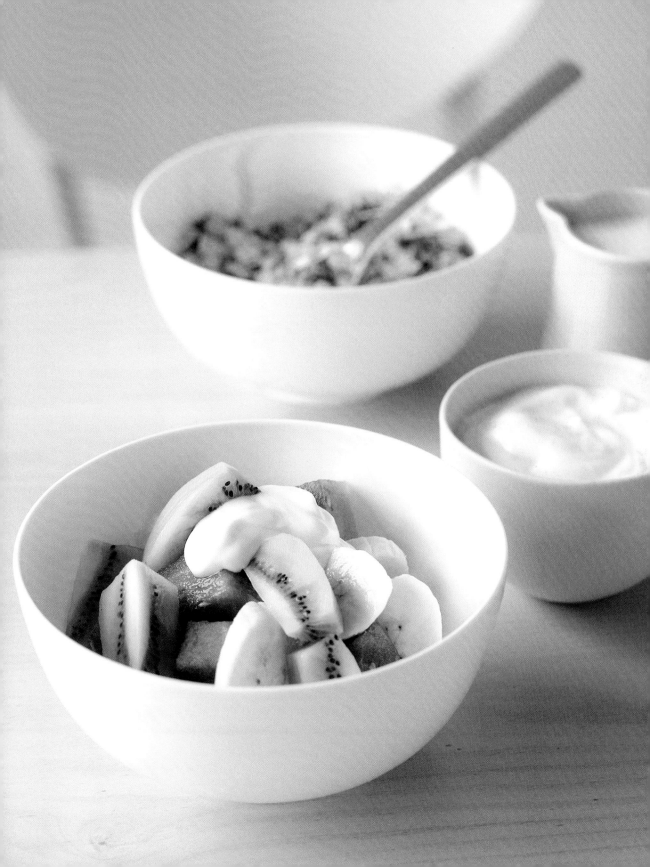

entrees

These meals can be prepared as lunches or dinners. Try to keep your lunches pretty generous—remember, eat breakfast like a king, lunch like a prince, and dinner like a pauper. The quantities I use here are to serve two, so adjust them up or down as required. It's always handy to have some leftovers to refrigerate for another meal. And don't panic if you don't have everything listed in my recipes. As long as you have the core ingredients, you can add whatever herbs or vegetables you like—just watch your calories.

pan-fried shrimp and scallops with orange and tomato

I love this one! Calories total around 260.

Serves 2

1 clove garlic, crushed
1/4 cup freshly squeezed orange juice
1½ tablespoons fresh lime juice
1 tablespoon extra-virgin olive oil
1 tablespoon chopped fresh basil
1 tablespoon finely chopped fresh flat-leaf parsley
Freshly ground black pepper
1 large handful baby arugula
1 orange, peeled, white pith removed, segmented
2 large tomatoes (or 4 plum tomatoes), chopped
Olive oil, for pan frying
6 scallops
6 jumbo shrimp, peeled and deveined
1 clove garlic, finely chopped

To make the dressing, combine the garlic, orange juice, lime juice, olive oil, basil, parsley, and pepper. Arrange the arugula on a platter and scatter the orange and tomato on top. Lightly oil a nonstick frying pan and cook the scallops and shrimp for 1–2 minutes each side (shrimp will take a little longer). Arrange over the arugula salad. Add the garlic to the pan and cook for 10 seconds. Pour the garlic and any juices over the salad with the dressing and serve.

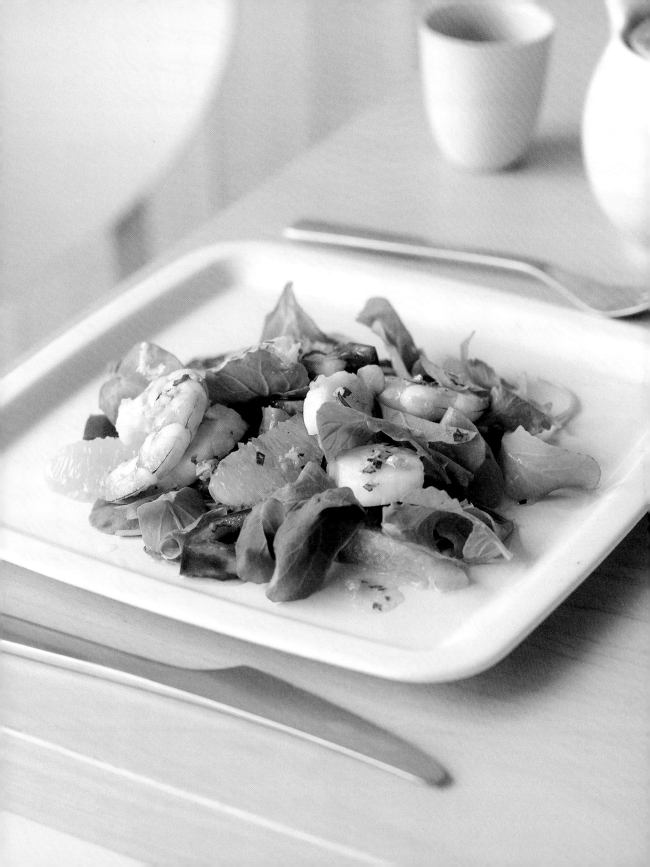

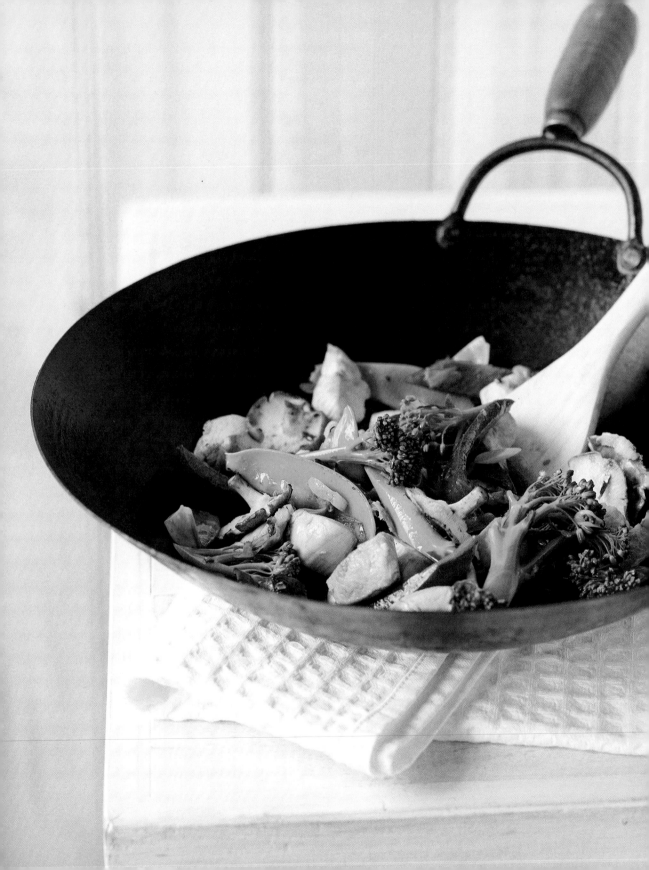

stir-fry

Stir-fries are a staple in my house. They are quick to prepare and nutritious, and the flavor combinations are endless. The secret to a good stir-fry is to have all of your ingredients prepared before you start and to keep the wok hot. I usually include five vegetables, three spices, and one protein ingredient (meat or tofu). For most of my combos, the calories add up to around 300.

Serves 2

Olive oil spray

10 oz meat or firm tofu, chopped into 3/4-inch cubes

1 small onion, peeled and quartered

2 cloves garlic, crushed

1 teaspoon finely grated fresh ginger

1 small red chile, seeded and finely chopped

10 oz mixed vegetables, washed and chopped

1 tablespoon soy or teriyaki sauce

2 tablespoons chopped fresh cilantro

Spray a nonstick wok with olive oil and heat until hot. Cook the meat or tofu, stirring constantly, for 2 minutes or until browned. The cooking time will vary depending on the type of meat. Remove and set aside in a bowl. Give the wok another light spray, brown the onion and garlic, then toss in the ginger, chile, and vegetables and cook for 2 minutes until tender but still crisp. Overcooked stir-fried veggies taste like crap, so keep them moving in the wok. Add the soy or teriyaki and the meat or tofu plus any juices, and cook for 1 minute. Serve garnished with cilantro.

Variations: Here are my favorite three key ingredients (protein/veggies/spices) in order of preference:

Protein: firm tofu, free-range chicken breast, shrimp, baby octopus

Veggies: onion, broccoli, baby bok choy, broccolini, red peppers, snow peas, Chinese mushrooms, scallions, asparagus, string beans, eggplant, baby corn

Spices/herbs: ginger, garlic, chiles, cilantro

salmon steak with arugula and asparagus

This is a favorite because it's quick, delicious, and only 300 calories. Get some nice Atlantic salmon, or you could use steelhead fillets (I prefer the middle cut but Billy finds it a bit too fatty, so he has the tail). Cooking time? About 7 minutes. And you wonder why I don't believe people when they tell me they don't have time to cook . . .

Serves 2

Olive oil spray

1 bunch fresh asparagus, trimmed

2 fresh salmon fillets, 5 oz each

Large handful baby arugula

½ red pepper, thinly sliced

Fresh dill fronds

Freshly ground black pepper

Spray a nonstick frying pan with olive oil and heat until hot. Pop in the asparagus and cook for 2–3 minutes; set aside and keep warm. Add the salmon fillets, skin side down, and cook for 3 minutes for rare and 4 minutes for well done. Turn them over and cook an additional 1 minute. Remove and serve on a bed of baby arugula with the red pepper and asparagus on the side. Garnish with dill and pepper.

Variation: Add chopped walnuts, thinly sliced fennel bulb, and chopped fennel leaves to the arugula salad.

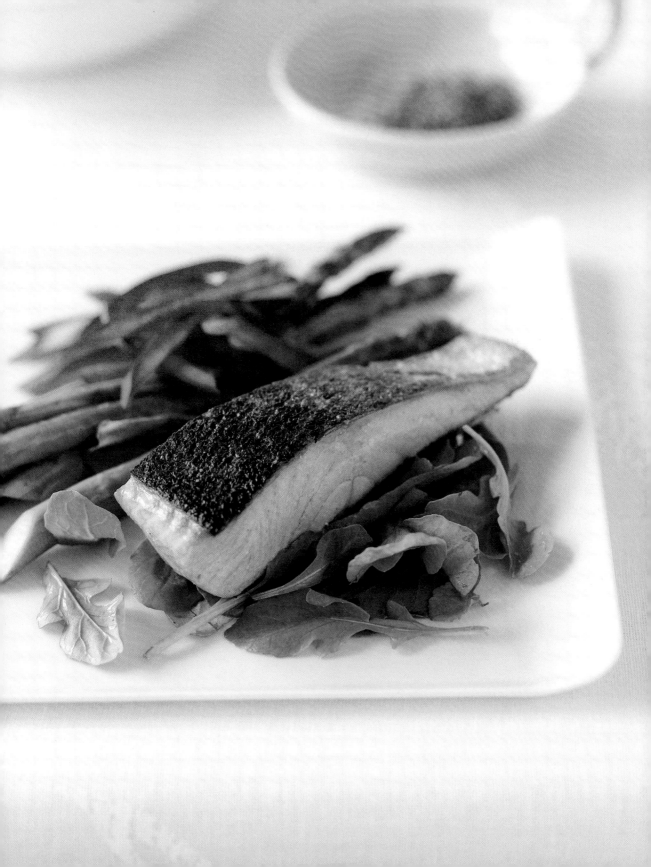

baked fish with eggplant

Add this to your list of "meals-that-cook-while-you're-in-the-shower" collection. It's also delicious and low in calories—around 300 per serving.

Serves 2

Olive oil, for pan-frying

1 onion, cut into thin wedges

½ medium eggplant, quartered and thinly sliced

3 tomatoes, chopped

1 teaspoon dried oregano

1 tablespoon drained capers

3–4 tablespoons low-fat plain yogurt

2 white fish fillets, 5 oz each

Lemon slices

Small fresh basil leaves

Preheat oven to 350°. Heat a little olive oil in a nonstick saucepan and cook the onion and eggplant for 5 minutes or until browned. Add the tomato and oregano, then cover and cook over low heat for 10 minutes.

Stir capers into the yogurt. Transfer the eggplant mixture to a baking dish, place the fish fillets on top, and spoon the yogurt mixture over the fish. Bake for 20–25 minutes or until fish flakes easily with a fork. Serve with lemon slices and fresh basil.

chicken drumsticks in tomato broth

This meal is so easy, and any leftovers are good to have cold the following day if you don't have a microwave handy. One serving is only 330 calories.

Serves 2

4 chicken drumsticks, skin removed

Olive oil, for pan frying

1 onion, thinly sliced

3 cloves garlic, crushed

1 can (15 oz) peeled tomatoes

1 6–8 oz package of button mushrooms, quartered

1 sprig fresh thyme

1 teaspoon dried oregano

4 oz green beans, trimmed, halved

Lightly oil a large saucepan. Add the drumsticks and cook until browned. Add all the remaining ingredients except the beans. Bring to a boil, then reduce the heat and simmer covered for 30 minutes or until the meat is falling off the bones. Add the beans and cook an additional 3 minutes or until tender.

Variation: For a more substantial meal, serve with brown rice, or with a side dish of steamed vegetables.

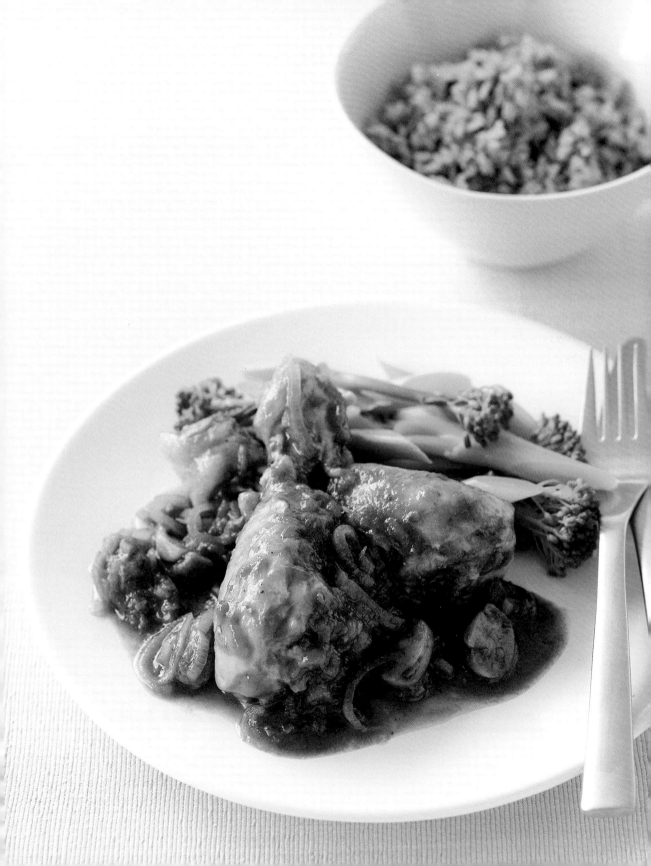

steamed fish and vegetables

This might sound plain, but it's a great dish and makes a light evening meal that fits the king, prince, pauper philosophy beautifully at around 375 calories per serving.

Serves 2

1 tablespoon lemon juice
2 tablespoons olive oil
1 clove garlic, finely chopped
1 scallion, thinly sliced on diagonal
1 teaspoon grated fresh ginger
2 white fish fillets, 5 oz each
1 carrot, julienned
2 ears corn
½ cup broccoli, cut into florets
1 lemon, cut into wedges for serving

Preheat the oven to 350°. Make a "tray" from aluminum foil, leaving enough on one side so that you can cover and seal the contents. Place the tray in a baking dish. Make up a marinade with the lemon juice, olive oil, garlic, scallion, and ginger. Place the fish fillets in the foil tray, pour the marinade over the top, and seal. Bake for 20–25 minutes, depending on the thickness of the fish. Meanwhile, steam the carrot (15 minutes), corn (10 minutes), and broccoli (5 minutes). Serve fish and vegetables together, drizzling the cooking juices over the top. Serve with lemon wedges.

Variation: Serve with other vegetables such as chayote squash (steam for 15 minutes), eggplant or mushrooms (5 minutes), and bok choy (3 minutes). I often serve the bok choy separately after marinating it in teriyaki sauce and sprinkling it with sesame seeds. You can also try steaming a whole trout in your wok, like the Chinese do. Get a wire rack that fits into your wok, leaving a little less than an inch underneath. Put the fish in a heatproof tray (you can buy foil trays at the supermarket), then mix 2 tablespoons light soy sauce with 2 tablespoons red wine vinegar, add some grated ginger, and pour it over the fish and leave to marinate for an hour or so. Fill the wok with water to just below the rack and bring it to a boil. Place the tray containing the fish on the rack. Sprinkle some finely sliced scallion, red peppers, and ginger on the fish, cover the wok, and steam for around 10–15 minutes, until tender.

vegetarian stack

As with all of my recipes, don't be constrained by my choice of veggies—add in anything you can bake. Because you're going to present it in a stack, you'll need the vegetables to be cut into large pieces. If you use the ingredients below, calories total around 360 per serving.

Serves 2

Olive oil spray

1 medium onion, cut into four 1/2-inch-thick slices

1 eggplant (about 1 lb), cut into four 1-inch-thick rounds

1 small-medium sweet potato, cut into four 1-inch-thick slices

2 large Portobello mushrooms, stems removed

½ red pepper, seeded and halved

1½ teaspoons chopped fresh rosemary

1 teaspoon ground cumin

1 teaspoon paprika

4 cloves garlic, peeled

½ bunch spinach, washed

1 cup low-fat ricotta cheese

Preheat the oven to 400°. Heat a nonstick frying pan sprayed with olive oil and brown the onion slices for 2 minutes on each side. (To keep them in one piece, use a spatula to move them.) Set aside. Steam the eggplant and sweet potato for 4 minutes or until slightly softened. Place in a lightly oiled baking dish with the onion, mushroom, and pepper and spray with olive oil. Mix together the rosemary, cumin, and paprika and sprinkle over the vegetables. Scatter the garlic cloves around and bake uncovered for 20–25 minutes, or until golden. Steam the spinach until just wilted. Place the mushrooms on 2 serving plates. Spread the garlic cloves over the mushrooms, then top with half the spinach, ricotta, eggplant, onion, pepper, and sweet potato. Repeat with remaining ingredients to make another layer, finishing with the sweet potato.

Tip: This meal is great with chutney or green tomato relish. Be careful, though—they can be very sugary.

penne with feta and lemon

This is a high-calorie meal, so I would never have it for dinner, only for lunch when I've either trained hard in the morning or have a big training session planned for that evening. This recipe makes enough for two medium servings, about 480 calories per serving.

Serves 2

2 cups penne pasta

1 teaspoon grated lemon zest

2 tablespoons lemon juice

2 tablespoons olive oil

1/2 cup crumbled low-fat feta

1 tablespoon pine nuts, toasted

1 tablespoon chopped fresh flat-leaf parsley

Cook pasta in boiling water according to package directions. Meanwhile combine lemon zest, juice, and olive oil in a jar and shake. Place cooked penne in serving bowl, crumble feta over the top, and toss with pine nuts, parsley, and dressing. Serve immediately.

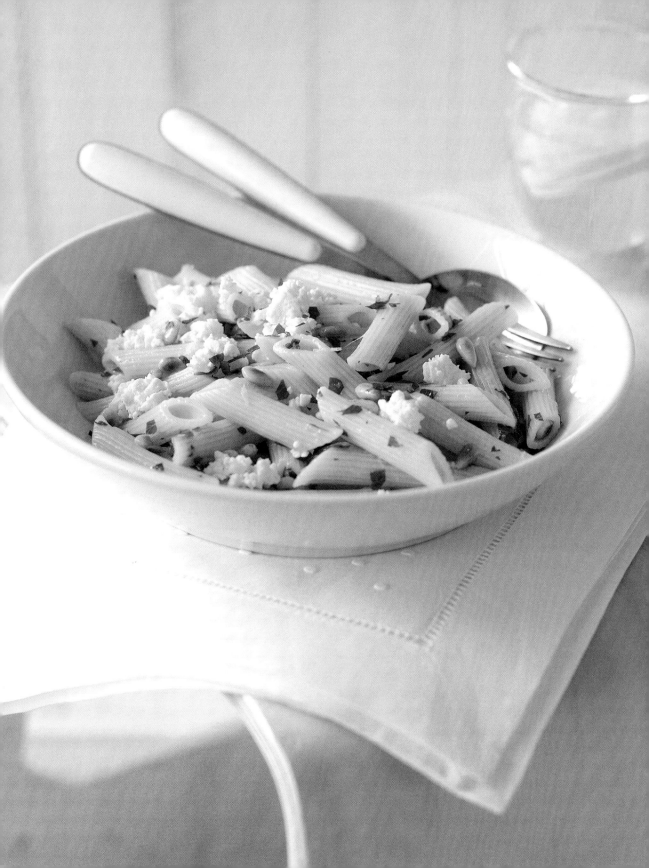

barbecued kebabs

The great thing about kebabs is that they're tricky to eat, which can slow you down and help you feel "full."
Be sure to soak the wooden skewers in water for an hour before cooking so they don't burn. We barbecue a lot
at home, but alcohol with barbecued food is strictly a treat. Have plain sparkling mineral water on hand with
a sprig of mint for hot summer days. All in, this one is around 120 calories per skewer.

Makes 8 skewers

1 red pepper, seeded and cut into
    sixteen 1-inch pieces
1 green pepper, seeded and cut into
    sixteen 1-inch pieces
8 button mushrooms, halved
1 zucchini, cut into sixteen ¼-inch rounds

16 cherry tomatoes
10 oz boneless chicken breast, cut into
    sixteen 1-inch cubes
1 red onion, cut into 8 wedges
Olive oil spray
Lemon wedges, for serving

Thread pieces of red and green peppers onto each skewer, then ½ mushroom, 1 zucchini round, 1 tomato, 1 piece chicken, 1 onion wedge, then another piece of chicken. Repeat with another tomato, zucchini, mushroom, and the peppers. Repeat to make 8 skewers. Spray with olive oil and cook on a preheated grill over medium heat for 12–15 minutes, turning to avoid burning. Serve with lemon wedges.

Variation: Marinate the chicken in olive oil, lemon juice, freshly ground black pepper, and chopped thyme for an hour before cooking. Or replace the chicken with shrimp or tofu and marinate in olive oil, thyme, chile, and garlic for 1–2 hours.

sides

These are my favorite sides. They are not too fancy, so it's easy to experiment.

barbecued vegetables

Why do we always associate barbecues with meat? They are great for cooking vegetables! Any leftovers will last in the fridge for a day or two. The veggies below total around 300 calories per serving.

Serves 2

1 onion, peeled and cut into wedges (if you don't cut off the end, it will help the wedges stay together)

1 large slender eggplant, thinly sliced lengthways

1 red pepper, cut into thick strips

1 zucchini, sliced lengthways

1 Portobello mushroom, thickly sliced

2 tablespoons olive oil

2 teaspoons chopped fresh rosemary

1 tomato, thickly sliced

Place the onion, eggplant, peppers, zucchini, mushroom, and oil in a bowl and toss to coat. Heat a grill or ridged grill pan over high heat and cook the vegetables for 4–5 minutes each side or until tender. (Put the peppers on first, as those take the longest to cook.) Add the tomato slices and cook for 1–2 minutes each side. Remove the vegetables, except the tomato, and toss with the rosemary. Serve topped with the tomato.

broccoli and cauliflower with paprika

A nice way to spice up some steamed veggies! Calories total around 120.

Serves 2

4 oz cauliflower, cut into bite-sized pieces
4 oz broccoli, cut into bite-sized pieces
Paprika, for dusting
Olive oil spray

Steam the cauliflower and broccoli until tender. Dust them with paprika. Lightly spray a nonstick frying pan with olive oil and place over high heat. Add cauliflower and broccoli and cook until heated through. Serve immediately.

bok choy in light soy with sesame seeds

Bok choy turns up a lot in my recipes. I love its peppery flavor, and it also happens to be very nutritious! This dish is around 120 calories.

Serves 1

1 bunch baby bok choy, washed and quartered, bottoms trimmed but intact
1 tablespoon light soy sauce
½ teaspoon sesame oil
1 tablespoon sesame seeds, toasted

Steam bok choy for 2–3 minutes or until tender. Transfer to a plate or serving dish. Mix together the soy sauce and sesame oil and pour over the bok choy. Sprinkle with sesame seeds and serve.

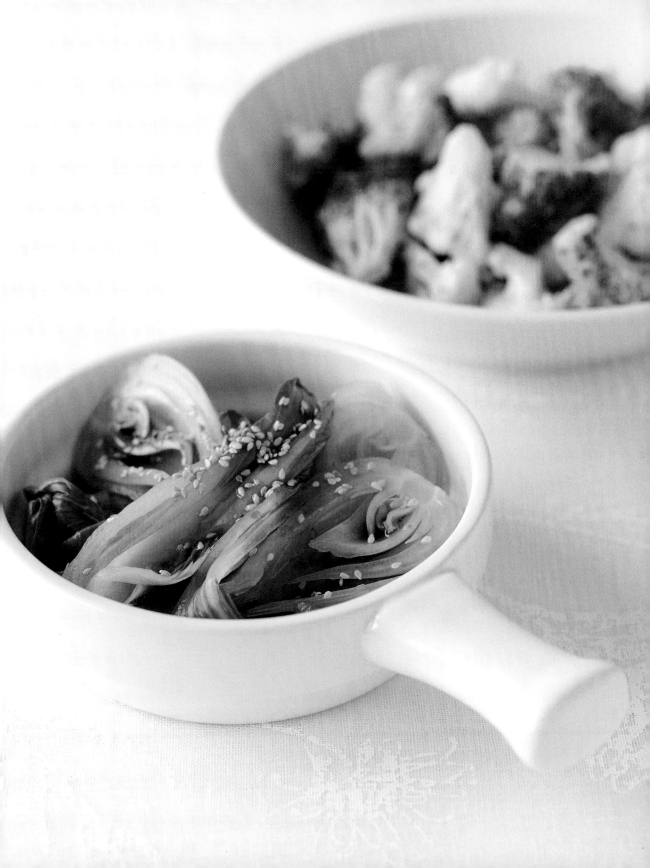

stuffed red peppers

Yum! This is a goodie that I often prepare when I've got the oven on and have an assortment of veggies that need to be used up. This one's around 200 calories per serving.

Serves 2

2 red peppers

Olive oil spray

1 small onion, chopped

1 tomato, chopped

1 Portobello mushroom, chopped

2 cloves garlic

1 teaspoon chopped fresh oregano (optional)

1 tablespoon pumpkin seeds (optional)

1 tablespoon sunflower seeds (optional)

1 tablespoon chopped fresh flat-leaf parsley
   (optional)

½ (15 oz) can crushed tomatoes

¼ teaspoon dried oregano

Freshly ground black pepper

Preheat oven to 350°. Cut the tops off the peppers and set aside. Remove the seeds and membranes and trim the base so they will stand upright. Put them in a saucepan of boiling water for 3 minutes to soften, and drain well. Spray a nonstick saucepan with olive oil, add the onion, and cook over medium heat for 2–3 minutes or until softened. Add the tomato, mushroom, and 1 clove finely chopped garlic and cook, stirring, for 4 minutes. Feel free to add fresh oregano, pumpkin seeds, sunflower seeds, and/or parsley at this point. Stuff the mixture into the blanched peppers, pop the little lids back on, and stand in an ovenproof dish with a little water in the bottom. Cover and bake for 40 minutes. Meanwhile, place the crushed tomatoes, 1 clove of crushed garlic, dried oregano, and pepper in the saucepan and stir to combine and heat through. Serve over the stuffed peppers.

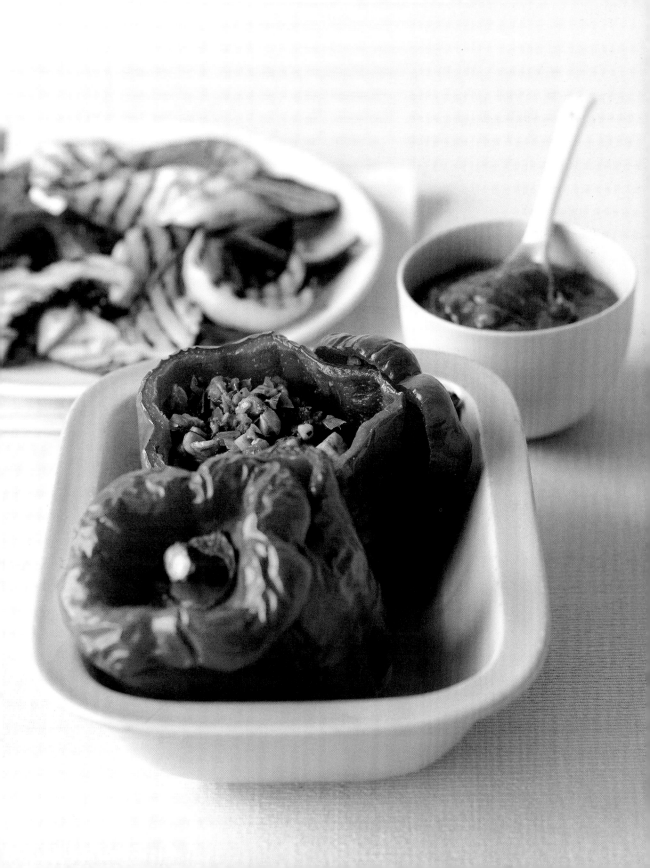

soups and salads

Anyone who is serious about weight management needs to be a master of salads. The great thing with salads is that there are no rules, really—keep the ingredients you like handy and add them to suit your mood.

Warning! You can eat salad greens and vegetables till the cows come home, but beware of calorie-dense ingredients such as olive oil, cheese, and nuts. For example:

- 1 whole walnut = around 25 calories
- 1 tablespoon Parmesan = around 50 calories
- 1 tablespoon pine nuts = around 80 calories
- 1 tablespoon olive oil = 120 calories
- 1 oz low-fat feta = 70 calories

vegetable soup

This is a winter favorite, and it freezes well, so make plenty of it for future meals. When reheating it you can also add some meat of your choice, or some extra leafy green vegetables. I often use all my leftover veggies, so it is different every time. The ingredients below will give you about 250 calories per serving.

Serves 4

1 cup brown lentils	1 quart reduced-salt vegetable stock
2 teaspoons olive oil	3 large carrots, peeled and sliced
1 leek (white part only), washed and finely chopped	1 parsnip, peeled and cut into ½-inch cubes
2 cloves garlic, crushed	6 Brussels sprouts, halved
4 bay leaves	1 medium zucchini, cut into ½-inch cubes
1 sprig fresh rosemary	Handful of green beans, trimmed, cut into 1-inch lengths

Pick over the lentils, rinse them in cold water, and drain. Heat the oil in a large saucepan and cook the leek for 4–5 minutes over medium heat until softened. Add the garlic and cook for 20 seconds. Add the lentils, bay leaves, rosemary, and stock and bring to a boil. Reduce the heat to low, cover, and cook for 1 hour or until lentils are tender. Add the carrots and parsnip and cook, covered, for 15 minutes, or until tender, adding water as necessary. Add the Brussels sprouts, zucchini, and beans and cook, covered, an additional 4 minutes, or until tender. Discard rosemary sprig and bay leaves.

Variation: Serve with some green leafy vegetables such as chard or quartered bok choy on top—the heat from the soup will be enough to cook them through after a couple of minutes.

leafy green salad

As a rule of thumb, I use four staple ingredients in my green salad and then add whatever bits and pieces I have around. I often buy the supermarket bags of mixed greens, which usually contain several types, such as arugula, radicchio, endive, and baby spinach. I always use cold-pressed extra-virgin olive oil for salads, as it tastes the best. This is around 220 calories.

Serves 2

4 oz mixed lettuce leaves

2 small tomatoes, quartered

1 seedless cucumber, quartered lengthways
    and sliced

6 button mushrooms, quartered

2 oz crumbled low-fat feta

1 tablespoon chopped fresh mint (or to taste)

freshly ground black pepper

1½ tablespoons cold-pressed extra-virgin olive oil,
    for drizzling

Combine all ingredients in a bowl except the oil. Add this *after* you've served it—that way you can keep the leftovers in the fridge without them going soft and brown.

Variations: If you like a bit more bite in your salad, add sliced scallions or replace the mint with basil. You can also sprinkle a few pumpkin seeds on top, or for a sweeter taste, try a few grapes or even strawberries. Experiment to find the flavors you like.

beet, feta, and walnut salad

This is a favorite of mine, though if you don't want your fingers stained pink from the beets, try wearing disposable rubber gloves when you handle them. Calories total 300, or 200 without the walnuts.

Serves 2

12 oz trimmed baby beets

1½ tablespoons cold-pressed extra-virgin
   olive oil

3 teaspoons red wine vinegar

Freshly ground black pepper

Large handful (40 g) baby arugula

4 oz low-fat feta, cubed

¼ cup walnut halves

Steam the beets for about 30–40 minutes or until soft, then peel, quarter, and allow to cool in a bowl. Mix together the oil, vinegar, and pepper and toss with the beets. Place the arugula in another bowl with the feta and walnuts. To avoid staining everything red, serve side by side rather than tossing together.

Note: When you really need to reduce calories, substitute the olive oil (1½ tablespoons is a whopping 180 calories) with lemon juice—this is what *The Biggest Loser* contestants always do.

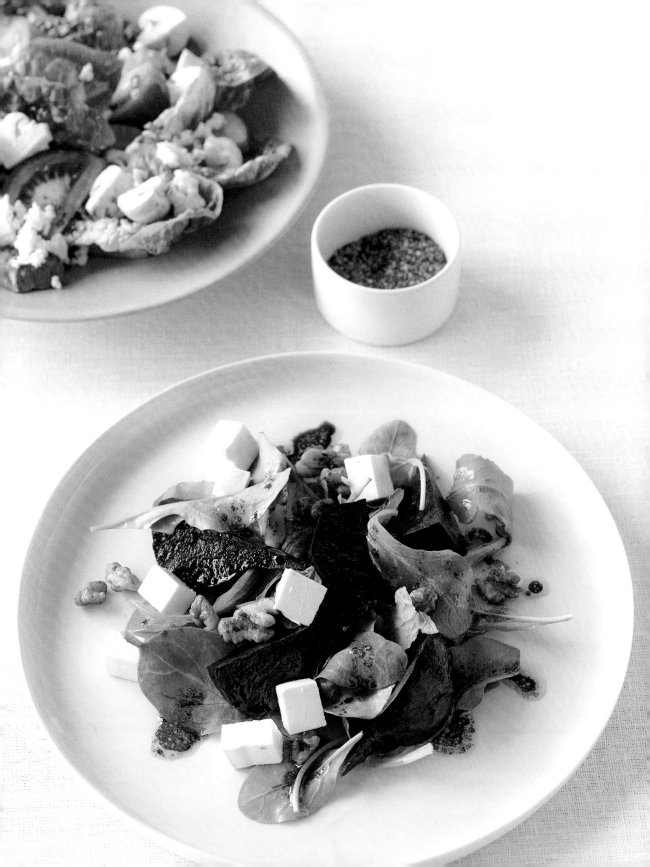

arugula and pear salad

This is so easy and really reminds me of summer. It's around 375 calories per serving, or 230 without the nuts.

2 handfuls baby arugula

1 ripe pear, cored and sliced

2 tablespoons shaved Parmesan or crumbled blue cheese

¼ cup pecans or walnuts

1 tablespoon cold-pressed extra-virgin olive oil

2 teaspoons lemon juice

Place the arugula in a salad bowl and top with the pear slices, cheese, and nuts. Mix together the olive oil and lemon juice and pour over the salad.

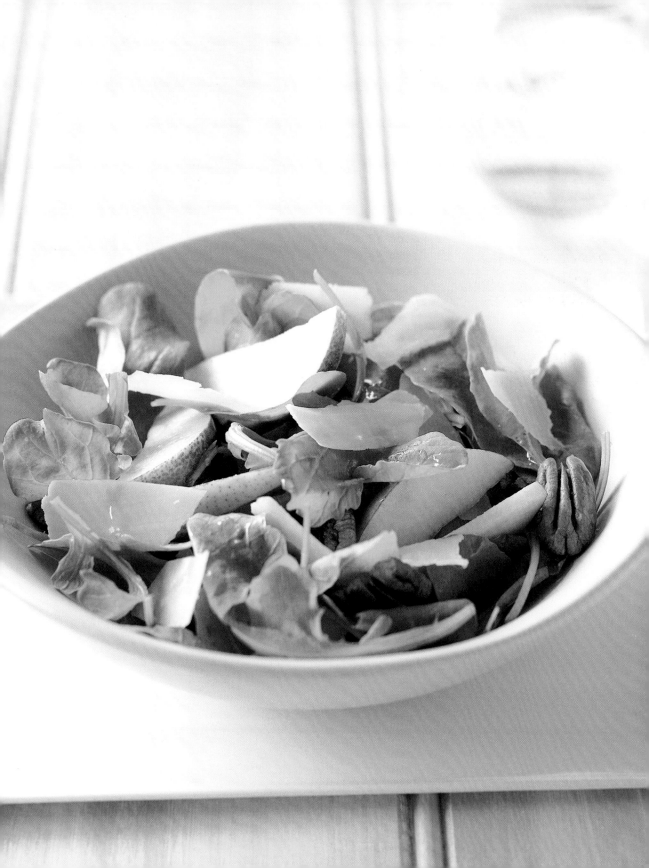

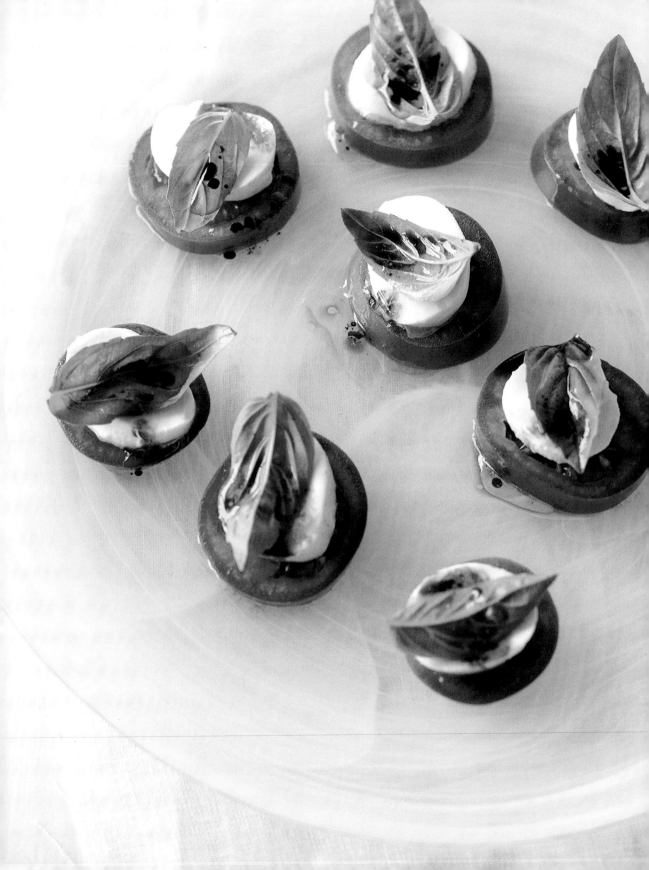

tomato, mozzarella, and basil stacks

One of my all-time faves! It's super quick, it's low in calories at 300 per serving, and it looks impressive, too.

Serves 2

2 large ripe plum tomatoes, cut into ½-inch-thick rounds

5 oz mozzarella, sliced into ½-inch-thick rounds

12 whole fresh basil leaves

1 tablespoon cold-pressed extra-virgin olive oil

2 teaspoons balsamic vinegar

Freshly ground black pepper

Arrange the tomato rounds in a single layer on a plate and top each one with a slice of mozzarella and a basil leaf. Combine the olive oil, vinegar, and pepper and drizzle over the stacks.

string bean salad

This fresh and crunchy salad is great with meat dishes. Calories add up to around 200 per serving.

Serves 2

8 oz green beans, trimmed

1 tablespoon pine nuts

¼ red onion, finely sliced

½ teaspoon finely grated lemon zest

½ cup cherry tomatoes, halved

1 tablespoon cold-pressed extra-virgin olive oil

1 teaspoon lemon juice

1 teaspoon balsamic vinegar

Place the beans in a saucepan of boiling water for 1–2 minutes, until just tender. Drain, then refresh in cold water. Toast the pine nuts in a dry frying pan for a few minutes (keep an eye on them, as they burn easily). Remove from heat and combine in a bowl with the beans, onion, lemon zest, and cherry tomatoes. Mix together the olive oil, lemon juice, and vinegar and drizzle over the salad.

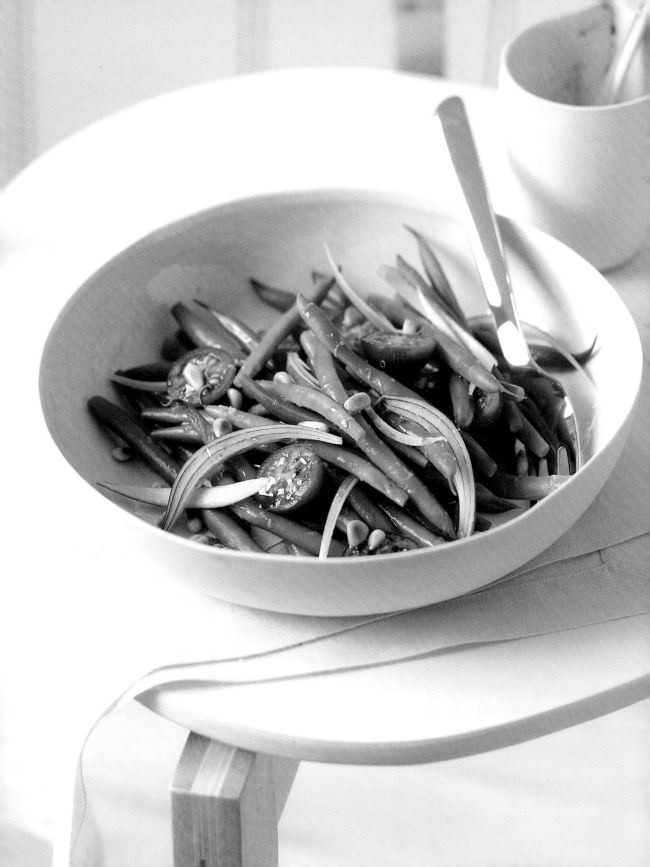

staying on track

Okay, so you've reached your goal weight. What happens now? First of all, you've got to be able to close the door on this part of your life and let it go. Let go of the overweight person you used to be, the history of unhappiness, the photos, the "fat" clothes—everything. That part of your life is finished. Love it and leave it. That's not who you are now.

But are you the kind of person who is able to set new goals and refocus? Or are you someone who goes off the rails once you've reached your target weight? I know plenty of people who do the latter—who fall in a heap without the imposed structure of their weight loss plans and stumble back into old habits.

Clearly, it is easier to stay motivated when you've set weight loss goals and you're actually *seeing* the scale readouts drop every week—nothing motivates like success. But how do you ensure that you keep the weight off? Trust me, there will come a time when there's just no motivation in the tank and you will feel the pull of old behavioral patterns (emotional eating, playing the victim, blaming others for not exercising). What then? Are you going to pack it in, give up, and go back to your old ways? *No!* That was the old you. The new you knows that exercising and healthy eating is simply something that you do. Just like you brush your hair and take a shower every day, you exercise and eat well every day. You know that it's no big drama—it's just what you *choose* to do in order to have a happy and fulfilling life.

So the day you step on the scale and hit your goal weight, you will give yourself a big pat on the back and be off to the gym, following it up with a healthful, nutritious meal. *It just doesn't stop. Ever.* Where you are right now and the things that you have learned about exercise, about nutrition, and about yourself are priceless. It's time for you to pay it forward. This is a gift you can pass on to your children, family, and friends. You are an inspiration to those around you because you have done what everyone seems to think is impossible.

So what are your next goals? Climbing a 14,000-foot mountain? Hiking in Nepal? There are no limits, especially when you look back at how far you have already come. Get out there and start truly living your life and sharing it with your family and friends. Isn't that what life is about, anyway?

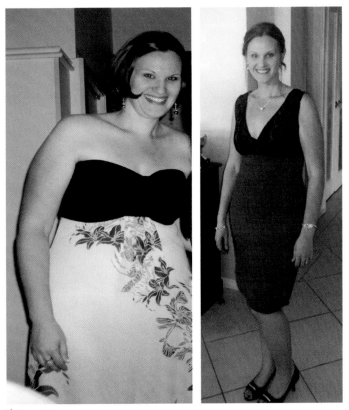

Mandy
Lost 45 pounds.

"Michelle's program has changed my life—I've recently become a fitness instructor."

"new you" journal

Here are simple versions of the templates I give my clients to record their progress. Copy them into your journal, or download them from my website, www.michellebridges.com.

daily food/exercise diary

food	calories In
breakfast	
snack (optional)	
lunch	
snack (optional)	
dinner	
	total

exercise	calories out
	basal metabolic rate
	total
	calorie surplus/deficit

physically I felt:

emotionally I felt:

weekly summary

	mon	tue	wed	thu	fri	sat	sun	total
calorie surplus/ deficit								

last week's weight   this week's weight   difference

12-week progress chart

	weight	calorie surplus/deficit	chest	waist	hips	thighs	arms
						measurements	
start							
week 1							
week 2							
week 3							
week 4							
week 5							
week 6							
week 7							
week 8							
week 9							
week 10							
week 11							
week 12							

blood pressure   cholesterol

Start   Week 12   Start   Week 12

acknowledgments

The sign on the front door of my office says "Michelle Bridges Team." I chose those words because it serves as a reminder of what I was once told by a Kahuna, a spiritual wise man, when I was in Hawaii one year. He told me that we should always remain humble because we only achieve things in life with the support and love of others.

This book is once again a great example of a lot of wonderful people pulling together and in doing so, achieving something special.

My thanks to Carl Fennessy and the Shine team, who got me started with my first series of *The Biggest Loser*. So much of this began with your belief in me all those years ago.

My amazing U.S. publishing team at Galvanized, David Zinczenko, and Steve Perrine, who made this happen in record time, and my gorgeous literary agent Celeste Fine. You guys rock! And talking of people who rock, Andrea Macnamara from Penguin Australia—thank you for nagging me!

The work behind the scenes is the glue that holds all this together—Stacey Navarro, Jackie Lann Brockman, Alora Alexander, and Jamie Krauss from The Narrative Group, Megan Hoelle, Colin Stewart, and the team at Blue State Digital, Anne McKevitt from The Million Dollar Plus Club who simply wouldn't take "no" for an answer. And to Michael Barry from Morrison Cohen, who kept us all legal.

To the amazing Henryk Lobaczewski and Alison Boyle, whose photography skills and hair and makeup artistry conspired so wonderfully to make me look younger. My stylist Lucia Arias-Martinez—thank you for your patience and vision.

To my friends and partners in the now world-renowned Michelle Bridges 12 Week Body Transformation online program, Tim and Amelia Phillips. OMG—your talents, belief, and dedication have contributed to the empowerment of hundreds of thousands of people. We're going to change the world!

I'm probably the only celebrity in the world whoactually loves her agent, but that's because she's fabulous! My thanks to the tireless Jane Weston and the Chic Celebrity team, and to Ursula Hufnagl and Pete O'Connell for their wisdom and belief. And to my friend Billy Moore, who's been with me on this journey from the start.

selected references

Training on Older Patients with Major Depression," *Archives of Internal Medicine,* October 25, 1999, cited in *Fitness and Nutrition: Exercise and Depression,* www.cvshealthresources.com/topic/exdepression (accessed April 2008).

Boutcher, S., G. Trapp, and Y. Boutcher, "Catecholamine and lactate response to high intensity intermittent cycle exercise," School of Medical Sciences, UNSW, reported in *Science Daily,* www.sciencedaily.com/releases/2007/02/0727185835.htm (accessed May 2008).

Cornforth, T., *Women's Health*, www.womenshealth.about.com/cs/gallbladder/a/dieting gallston_2.htm (accessed March 2008).

Drago, L. et al., "Diabetes and Nutrition: Carbohydrates," *Journal of Clinical Endocrinology and Metabolism,* vol. 93, no. 3, March 1, 2008, http://jcem.endojournals.org/cgi/content/full/93/3/0 (accessed June 2008).

International Food Information Council, "Dietary Fats and Fat Replacers," *IFIC Foundation Media Guide on Food Safety and Nutrition*, 2007–2009, http://ific.org (accessed July 2008).

Pavlou, K. N. et al., "Effects of Dieting and Exercise on Lean Body Mass, Oxygen Uptake and Strength," *Medicine and Science in Sports and Exercise,* vol. 17, no. 4, August 1985.

Toouli, J., interviewed for media release "Rapid Weight Loss Linked to Gallstones," Department of Surgery, Flinders Medical Center, April 2, 2002, www.flinders.sa.gov.au/research/files/links/GallstonesResearch.pdf.

index

A

abdominal training, 99–107
aerobic (cardio) training, 60–1
    circuit training, 62–3, 133, 134, 137
    group fitness classes, 60, 63
    interval training, 62
    jogging, 41, 60, 113, 114
    maximum heart rate (MHR), 62, 75
    plyometric exercises, 63
    12-week program, 133–65
    See also fitness training
agility training, 119
alcohol
    alcoholic beverages, 181–2
    as carbohydrate, 171, 172, 173, 175
arms and shoulders
    measuring arms, 27
    toning exercises, 96–8

B

back stretch, 127
back toning exercises, 86–9
back twist, 127
bad habits, 15–16, 22
basal metabolic rate (BMR), 11, 35, 38, 40
"benchmark clothes," 27
The Biggest Loser, 21, 27, 44, 62, 75, 113, 165, 177, 183, 191
BMI. *See* body mass index
BMR. *See* basal metabolic rate
body
    muscles, 64, 76
    self-hate, 25–6
body mass index (BMI), 27, 35–6
    calculating, 35
    gallstones and, 57
    height/weight chart, 49
    meaning of BMI numbers, 36
body measurements, 26–7, 32

BodyAttack, 63
BodyBalance, 63, 135
BodyPump, 63, 136
boxing, 126, 136
breakfast, 170, 180, 182, 190, 192, 195
breakfast cereal, 170
breakfast recipes, 195–200
    cottage or ricotta cheese on toast, 196
    egg-white omelette with toast, 196
    fruit and yogurt, 200
    homemade muesli with yogurt, 200
    oatmeal, 199
    poached egg on toast, 199

C

calendar, planning weight loss, 27–8
calf stretch, 130
calorie counter, 27
calorie counting, 27, 32, 44, 170, 179, 181, 189–91
calorie deficit, 44
calorie-dense foods, 171, 172, 180
calorie expenditure
    chart, 41
    exercise and, 37, 40–4
calorie intake, 32, 37–8, 179, 189–91
calories
    burning, 37–8, 40–4
    daily calorie quota, 179, 189–91
    intake, 32, 37–8, 179, 189–91
    portion size and, 179
    sample eating plan, 192–3
    in snacks, 37, 170, 179, 192–3
calories in-calories out equation, 37
carbohydrate-rich foods, 172
carbohydrates, 171, 172
    alcohol, 171, 172, 173, 175
    rate of digestion, 11
    weight loss and, 63–4

cardio training. *See* aerobic (cardio) training; fitness training
cereals, 170
cheese, 12, 220
chest measurement, 26
chest stretch, 130
chest toning exercises, 90–5
child's pose (stretch), 129
chocolate treat, 190
circuit training, 62–3, 133, 134, 137
compound exercises, 74
cooking, 176, 182–3, 195
    See also recipes
core toning
    exercises, 99–107
    stretches following, 135
    12-week program, 133–65
cortisol, 13
crunches, 99–102
cycling, 41, 60, 118

D

daily calorie expenditure, thermal effect of food, 11
daily journal, 31
    See also journal of "the new you"
denial, 17–18
depression, exercise and, 53
diaries and journals. *See* daily journal; food diary; journal of "the new you"
diet
    alcoholic beverages, 181–2
    calorie counting, 27, 32, 44, 170, 179, 181, 189–91
    calorie intake, 32, 37–8, 179, 189–91
    fats in, 56–7, 172, 173
    low-calorie diet, 56, 68–9, 190, 191
    "low-fat" foods, 170, 180, 181
    portion control, 178–9

diet (*cont.*)

    sample eating plan, 192–3

    snacks, 37, 170, 179, 180, 182, 192–3

    See also eating; food; meals

digestion, rate of, 11

dinner, 182–3, 190, 193, 202

    entree recipes, 202–14

    salad and soup recipes, 220–8

    side dish recipes, 215–18

drinking alcoholic beverages, 181–2

drinking water, 10–11, 56

dumbbell weight, guide, 134

E

eating

    eating regularly, 10, 56–7, 175–6, 179–80

    "low-fat" trap, 170, 180, 181

    portion control, 178–9

    rate of digestion and, 11–12

    reward syndrome, 57, 60, 65

    sample eating plan, 192–3

    skipping meals, 189–90

    snowball theory, 187

    See also diet; food; recipes

eating plan

    calories, 189–91

    day by day plan, 192–3

    plan for, 190

    See also recipes

emotional relationship with food, 169

emotions, daily journal, 31

"enrollment conversation," 29, 31

entree recipes, 202–14

    baked fish with eggplant, 208

    barbecued kebabs, 214

    chicken drumsticks in tomato broth, 208

    pan-fried shrimp and scallops with orange and tomato, 202

    penne with feta and lemon, 212

    salmon steak with arugula and asparagus, 206

    steamed fish and vegetables, 210

    stir fry, 205

    vegetarian stack, 211

EPOC. *See* post-exercise oxygen consumption

equipment checklist, 77

excuses, 3, 5, 6, 15–17

    games with food, 179–80

    negative self-talk, 6, 18–19, 22, 55, 58–9

    no time, 28, 48

    reward syndrome, 57, 60, 65

    types of excuses, 16–17

exercise

    benefits, 7, 13, 53

    calorie expenditure, 37, 40–4

    calorie expenditure chart, 41

    depression and, 53

    excuses for not doing, 15–17

    formal vs. informal, 60

    group fitness classes, 60, 63

    intensity, 48, 61, 75

    low-intensity vs. high intensity, 48

    metabolism and, 12–13

    motivation, 20, 27, 231

    myths about fitness, 47–51

    side effects, 13, 55

    See also toning (weight training); training

exercises

    compound exercises, 74

    golden rules for, 77

    isolation exercises, 74–5

    plyometric exercises, 63

    rhythm changes, 78

    See also fitness training; flexibility training; toning (weight training)

F

facing fears, 7

family

    "enrollment conversation," 29, 31

    support of, 29

fast food, 170

fat

    losing fat during weight loss, 54, 73–4

    spot-reducing, 50

fats

    dietary, 56–7, 172, 173

    good and bad fats, 174

    hydrogenated, 174

    "low-fat" foods, 170, 180, 181

    mono-unsaturated, 174

    polyunsaturated, 174

    rate of digestion, 11

    saturated, 174

    trans fats, 174

fear of change, 7

fear of exercise, 7

fear of failure, 7

females

    daily calorie quotas, 179, 189

    getting big with weight training, 50–1

fiber, rate of digestion, 11

fish, health benefits, 12

fitness, myths about, 47–51

fitness class, calorie expenditure, 41

fitness days, workout program, 134

fitness training, 113

    agility training, 119

    boxing, 126, 136

    cycling, 41, 60, 118

    ice skaters on the spot, 121

    jogging, 41, 60, 113, 114

    jumping, 63, 120, 122–4

    jumping jacks, 123

    jumping rope, 118

    rowing machine, 118

    running, 61, 113–17

    See also aerobic (cardio) training

flexibility training, 60, 65, 126–7

    importance of, 127

    stretching exercises, 127–30

food

    alcohol as carb, 171, 172, 173, 175

    alcoholic beverages, 181–2

    before exercising, 49

    breakfast, 170, 180, 182, 190, 192, 195

    calorie counting, 27, 32, 44, 170, 179, 181, 189–91

    calorie-dense foods, 171, 172, 180

    calorie intake, 32, 37–8, 179, 189–91

    carbohydrates, 11, 63–4, 171, 172

    for celebration, 169

    components, 171

    cook the right stuff, 176

    creativity in cooking, 182–3

    daily journal, 31

    dinner, 182–3, 190, 193, 202

    eating healthy, 184

about the author

MICHELLE BRIDGES has worked in the fitness industry for over twenty years as a professional trainer and group fitness instructor. Her role in Australia's version of the hit reality show *The Biggest Loser*, combined with her highly successful online exercise and mind-set program, the 12 Week Body Transformation, has already connected her with hundreds of thousands of Australians, making her the country's most recognized and influential fitness personality. Now she's ready to take on America, bringing her passion for health and fitness and motivational message with her. Michelle's books include *Crunch Time, Crunch Time Cookbook, Losing the Last 5 Kilos, 5 Minutes a Day, The No Excuses Cookbook, Everyday Weight Loss, Your Best Body, Get Real!*, and *Superfoods Cookbook*.

michellebridges.com

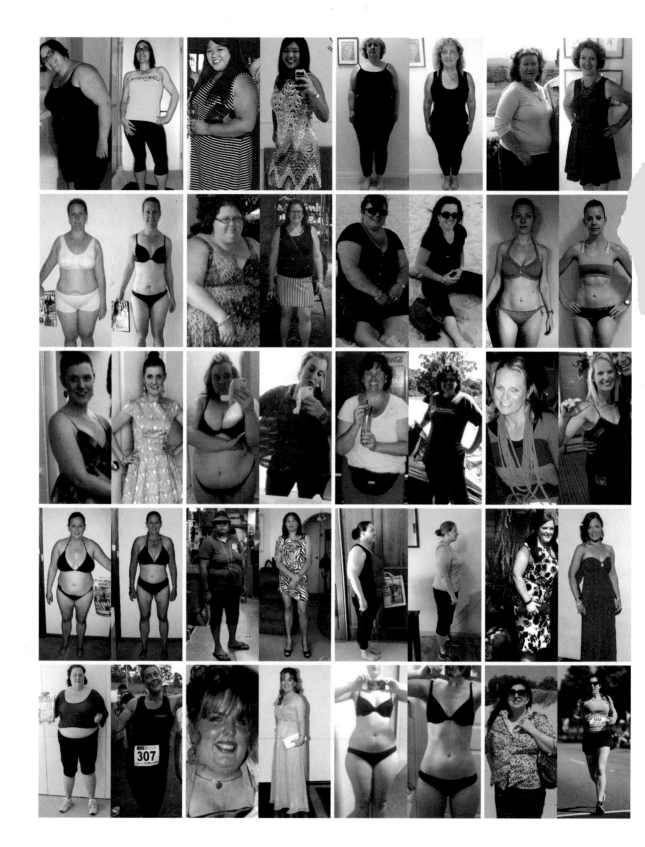